TAKE HEART!

A PROVEN STEP-BY-STEP PROGRAM TO IMPROVE YOUR HEART'S HEALTH

DR. TERENCE KAVANAGH

AUTHOR OF 'THE HEALTHY HEART PROGRAM'

KEY PORTER BOOKS

Canadian Cataloguing in Publication Data

Kavanagh, Terence
  Take heart

ISBN 1-55013-377-2

1. Coronary heart disease - Prevention.
2. Heart - Diseases - Patients - Rehabilitation.
I. Title.

RC685.C6K38 1992   616.1'2305   C92-093656-3

Key Porter Books Limited
70 The Esplanade
Toronto, Ontario
Canada M5E 1R2

Distributed in the United States of America by:
Publishers Group West
4065 Hollis
Emeryville, CA 94608

Illustrations and diagrams: Pages Design
Typesetting: True To Type Inc.

Printed and bound in Canada

92 93 94 95 96 6 5 4 3 2 1

Contents

Dedication

To the staff of the Toronto Rehabilitation Centre's Cardiac Department, whose dedication, loyalty, and hard work is a constant inspiration to me and to their patients.

Preface

My aim in writing this book is two-fold. Firstly, to help the layperson understand the nature of coronary heart disease, its causes, treatment, and prevention. Secondly, to emphasize the importance of regular physical activity in attaining and maintaining heart health.

These were the same aims that I had in 1968 when I started the Toronto Rehabilitation Centre's Cardiac Exercise Rehabilitation Program. Since then the program has grown in size and stature. With more than 1,000 new patient referrals each year, it is one of the largest, if not the largest of its type in the world. Of course, growth is not the only measure of success. More to the point is the fact that our approach has found favor with similar programs in North America, the United Kingdom, Italy, Australia, New Zealand, South Africa, and Singapore.

The following pages embody the Toronto program's concepts, methods, and extensive experience, and are directed not only to those who are suffering from coronary heart disease and do not have access to a physician-supervised formal exercise program, but also to those who are still healthy, and want to avoid a heart attack in the future. Needless to say, a guide such as this is meant as a complement to, rather than as a substitute for, your doctor's advice. Used in that context, I believe it can make a valuable contribution to your health and well-being.

Since this book is in large part the product of a highly viable and successful program, I would be remiss if I did not thank those "founding members" who helped me set it up and who are still actively involved: Johanna Kennedy, R.N.; Robin Campbell, B.P.H.E., M.S.; Salah Qureshi, B.Sc.; and Professor Roy Shephard, M.D., Ph.D., D.P.E.

No one person, and no group, operates in a vacuum. The Toronto Rehabilitation Centre is a public hospital. To its Board of Directors goes the credit for encouraging me, as Medical Director, and my staff in our efforts to institute an exercise program for heart patients.

It is, I know, customary for some health workers and physicians to criticize government-controlled medicine. Be that as it may, the Centre's operating funds are provided entirely by the Ontario Ministry of Health, and although over the years and from time to time we have had to endure necessary budgetary constraints, I have found the system to be fair and equitable. It has allowed us to provide the best possible service to our patients, and there can be no better testimonial than that.

As the program has grown, so has our need for additional space and equipment. In 1980 we opened a new two-storey wing, which included a 120-seat lecture theater for patients and their spouses, a large gymnasium, two exercise test laboratories, and a 200-meter walking/jogging track. The capital funding for this was raised by our charitable fund-raising organization, Marina Lodge, which consists mostly of present and past patients; I am deeply thankful for their efforts. This year, 1992, we are adding a 200-meter indoor track with additional space for patient monitoring and seminar rooms. Once again, all funding is being provided by Marina Lodge.

There are two essential ingredients to any successful

medical rehabilitation program: the patients, and the physicians who refer them. My heartfelt thanks to both. I always look upon any referral as both a compliment and an act of faith.

There is another group to which I feel a deep sense of obligation. Over the years, our patients' spouses and families have been our most ardent supporters. As is inevitable in any long-term follow-up program for heart attack patients such as ours, we must experience the reality of fatal recurrence, sometimes in those we have known for many years. In these circumstances, the relatives have gone out of their way to thank the program for helping to ensure that those final years were savored with zeal and enthusiasm. If nothing else, it is that attitude which makes our task one of the most satisfying in all of medicine.

Finally, this book would never have seen the light of day had it not been for my secretary, Janet Will, who typed the entire manuscript. She has endured long hours, countless delays on my part, and innumerable day-to-day frustrations, all with considerable patience and great tact. She has my sincerest thanks and respect.

1. A Modern Plague

Coronary heart disease has been called the twentieth-century plague. In 1990 the World Health Organization announced it to be our number-one killer. But despite this recent attention, the disease is not new. Examination of Egyptian mummies shows that it existed during the time of the pharaohs, 3,000 years ago. Greek and Roman literature contains many references to what sound suspiciously like fatal heart attacks, that is, sudden death after the onset of severe chest pain. During the sixteenth and seventeenth centuries, after the Church lifted the ban against autopsies and they became the recognized method of determining the cause of death, more and more deaths were attributed to what we recognize today as coronary heart disease (CHD).

William Heberden, the English physician, was the first to describe a symptom we now know to be an early manifestation of heart disease. Some of his patients, he said, "are seized while they are walking (more especially if it be uphill, and soon after eating) with a painful and most disagreeable sensation in the chest, which seems as if it would extinguish life if it were to increase or to continue; but the moment they stand still, all this uneasiness vanishes."

He called this symptom angina pectoris (Latin; pain in the chest), and both the name and the description of the symptom have been used by doctors ever since. Although Heberden was unable to explain the precise cause of the symptom, he realized that it was associated with some form of heart disorder. Throughout his long life — and he lived until the age of 91 — he faithfully recorded in detail each case he encountered. The fact that he accumulated only 100 such cases indicates that the condition was still relatively rare in the eighteenth century. Over the next hundred years, the theory slowly emerged that angina pectoris was caused by a disease process that *narrowed* the coronary arteries, the blood vessels that nourish the heart.

It was not until the early twentieth century that a Chicago physician, Dr. James Herrick, suggested that a heart attack was a later manifestation of the same process that caused angina pectoris, and that the heart attack was due to a *blockage* of a coronary artery. Herrick later commented on the fact that the scientific paper in which he first described this concept, published in 1912, aroused little interest among his fellow physicians at the time. Apparently in those days heart attacks were of less concern to doctors than they are today.

Currently, on a daily basis, heart attacks are responsible for some 2,000 deaths in the United States, 500 in the United Kingdom, and 250 in Canada. Approximately half these deaths occur in a matter of hours after the onset of chest pain, and before the patient reaches hospital. Three out of four victims are male and under the age of 55. In the United States, in addition to the three-quarters of a million people who suffer non-fatal heart attacks annually, more than 6 million have symptoms of coronary heart disease, and it is estimated that nearly 70% of adult Americans have some degree of narrowing of the coronary arteries. Initially a scourge of the Western industrialized countries, coronary heart disease is now also devastating the developing nations. There are few of us today who do not have a relative or friend who has fallen victim to this disease.

How did all this come about? It was once thought that the epidemic was more apparent than real, that doctors were simply diagnosing the cause of death with greater accuracy than their predecessors. Further investigation and observations on an international scale dispelled this theory and confirmed that heart attack mortality was on the increase. What had changed? Was it the population, the disease, or the environment? There is no evidence that human biology has changed, only a slight possibility that the disease has altered, and a good deal of evidence that it is our increasingly affluent lifestyle that is at fault. We will explore all of this later. In the meantime, let us take a closer look at the villain of the piece, known medically as a myocardial infarction, more commonly referred to as a heart attack.

PROFILE OF A HEART ATTACK VICTIM

John S. was entitled to feel pleased with himself. A professional engineer, at 41 he possessed all the contemporary hallmarks of success: a happy marriage, two teenaged boys who were doing well at school, a comfortable house (almost paid for) in a desirable neighborhood, and the prospect of promotion to company vice-president. Mind you, he hadn't had too much time of late to count his blessings; a year previously the company plant started moving to a new location, and as production manager, he had found himself involved in a hectic work schedule. Even Mary, his usually patient wife, began to express concern as six- and seven-day work weeks became routine. Still, the job had to be done, and as he said, "Goodness only knows what a mess things would get into if I wasn't there to keep tabs on everything." Besides, when the move was completed, he could ease off a bit, maybe "play a little golf, or take a week's vacation and get in a little fishing." Maybe he would cut back on his smoking, too; with all the stress, he was up to a pack and a half a day now. It wouldn't do any harm to lose a little weight also, but that was difficult when one's meals consisted of an endless succession of hurried sandwiches interspersed with "two-martini luncheon meetings" and expense-account dinners.

Yes, he probably was a little out of shape — which no doubt accounted for the heartburn and indigestion pain he had begun to experience in recent months whenever he got uptight at work or tried to lift anything heavy. He thought perhaps he was developing a peptic ulcer, the almost prestigious occupational disease of successful executives.

In due course, John's plant completed its move. But the transition brought with it problems that, naturally, only John could solve. Admittedly, weekends at the office were no longer routine (although they did occur from time to time), but the 12- and 13-hour workday became commonplace. Always a hard driver, he was now hotly in pursuit of the presidency, and he dedicated himself to the task with all the energy and determination that had characterized his performance as one of the best linemen of his university football team. Unfortunately, he wasn't in his early twenties any more and, while he still possessed the spirit and motivation of bygone years, his body was no longer fit enough to perform the tasks he asked of it. His "indigestion" pain was bothering him more frequently now, and not only after eating. From time to time, he experienced severe discomfort in his upper abdomen and chest when he ran up a flight of stairs, or walked quickly up an incline (not that he did too much walking nowadays). Usually, the pain would go away if he belched or rested for a minute or so.

He began to feel chronically tired. Never at any time, however, did he feel that he had any serious health problem. He always came through the annual company medical examination with flying colors; blood pressure, electrocardiogram, blood and urine checks always normal — which was, after all, only to be expected in a strong, tall ex-college football player.

Then one day, while sitting dozing in front of the television set, he got a fright; the stomach pain came on quite suddenly. Only on this occasion it was more severe and seemed to have moved up into his chest. For a moment or two, he had difficulty breathing, as the pain radiated first into his neck and jaw, and then down both arms to his hands. He found he was sweating profusely. He didn't know what to do. When he tried to lie down, the pain seemed to get worse; moving around didn't do any good, and neither did belching. Mary, noticing his agitation and pale, sweating features, learned for the first time of his recurrent bouts of "indigestion." She wanted to call a doctor, but John persuaded her to wait and see if his condition improved. Fortunately (or unfortunately, as it turned out), the pain subsided after about 30 minutes, although for the next day or two his chest felt very sore. In deference to Mary's wishes, he called his family physician the following week and told him that he had been getting "the occasional niggling stomach pain when I am overtired or tense." A combination of John's natural tendency to downplay any evidence of physical weakness, together with what may have been a too-easy acceptance of his tale by the physician, led to a diagnosis of "nerves." An electrocardiogram was not carried out.

During the following weeks, John continued his heavy work schedule, suffering only occasional and relatively mild "nerve" pains in his chest — until the week the plant workers went on strike. If the job was hectic before, it was frenetic now. Extra duties, extra hours, unpleasantness on the picket lines, all contributed to a desperate situation. There seemed to be no solution. As a matter of fact, there was, and in John's case, it was almost the final one.

At four o'clock one morning, he was awakened by the most severe pain in his chest he had ever experienced. It was as if a terrible weight was pressing on his chest bone, squeezing and squeezing until he felt he could no longer breathe. He thought he was going to die. He put up no argument when Mary called the ambulance. Within half an hour, an electrocardiogram was carried out in the emergency department and the young, serious-looking doctor quietly gave him the news; he had sustained a severe heart attack and was to be admitted to the intensive care unit immediately.

John was four weeks in hospital, during which time he experienced a series of emotional reactions to his predicament. At first, he was stunned by the doctor's diagnosis. It was impossible for him to have had a heart attack; his heart wasn't weak, he had never had a day's illness in his life — there must be some mistake. This period of denial lasted about 48 hours. Some patients never pass beyond it, even after discharge from hospital, persisting in their belief that the doctors have made a mistake. In John's case, it was replaced by a sullen anger. What right had fate to treat him in this unfair fashion? Hadn't he worked hard to make his mark in life, to provide for his wife and family, to get on? What reward was this for living according to the rules?

After he came out of intensive care, his cardiologist told him he would probably be able to go home in a couple of weeks. Always a stickler for accuracy, John interpreted "a couple" as being exactly two. When these two weeks were up, he was told he might be in hospital for another few weeks. He now became dreadfully depressed. He felt the doctors were keeping something from him; he was going to die, or at best he would be an invalid for the rest of his life.

Finally, John went home. He was still in a depressed mood. The first day back in familiar surroundings was almost too much for him. He felt so fatigued he had to go to bed after only a few hours. He had lost his old aggressive self-confidence and was fearful of responsibility. Even after his return to work, ostensibly fully recovered, Mary was at first surprised and then perturbed to find that he continued to lean on her, reluctant to take the initiative in financial or domestic matters requiring a decision.

This state of affairs continued until his doctor, sensing a deterioration in the family relationship, had a talk with him and asked him if he would like to attend an exercise rehabilitation class that had recently been instituted at the Toronto Rehabilitation Centre (TRC). John agreed. Later, he commented that the rehabilitation program was "like a lifebelt to a drowning man. It's the best thing since sliced bread."

Of course, there is no such thing as a typical heart attack victim. Patients come in all shapes, sizes, and types. John's story is a composite case history, drawn from the files of patients referred to the TRC for postcoronary rehabilitation. Interestingly, an analysis of these patients, published in the *Canadian Medical Journal*, revealed a surprising similarity in the patterns of life prior to their heart attacks. Comparison with a matched group of healthy individuals showed that the patients who had sustained a heart attack also experienced a greater than average degree of business, financial, or domestic stress in the year prior to their illness. In many cases, the stress factor was extreme.

In the last few weeks before the attack, a significant number of them had experienced vague pains in the chest, neck, jaw, or arms, but had ignored these symptoms, ascribing them to indigestion or nerves. Most described a feeling of incredible fatigue, one man actually falling asleep while dining with a business client, and another instinctively reacting to the news of his heart attack with the thought, "At least I'll be able to get a good sleep at the hospital." Overweight, heavy smoking, and lack of regular physical activity were all too common.

Often the attack itself occurred within 24 hours of a severe emotional experience or unaccustomed physical stress — for example, following a violent argument with the boss, or after half an hour of trying to start a stalled outboard motor. In at least one case, the emotional and physical were combined when a patient undertook a long and exhausting journey to see a boyhood house full of bittersweet memories.

Another study carried out at the TRC, also published in the *Canadian Medical Journal*, showed that many of these patients go through a phase of denial after the infarction, then all too frequently become depressed, lacking in confidence, and fearful for the future. The men feel they have lost their masculinity, and they worry about their ability to perform the role of husband and father with the same success as previously. Women victims feel a similar sense of insecurity, whether they are housewives or breadwinners. Both men and women hide their depression, even from their spouses, and it requires careful questioning by the physician and the psychologist to uncover it. Where depression exists, however, it is always profound.

By now you should be getting a picture of the manner in which coronary artery disease can strike its victim, often nowadays an apparently healthy, busy man in his forties. Women are less frequently affected, and we will see the reason for this later. But what exactly is coronary artery disease, and what causes it? In order to answer these questions, we must take a brief look at the anatomy and physiology of the heart and blood vessels, and then make a short excursion into the field of epidemiology.

THE HEART: STRUCTURE AND FUNCTION

Situated in the center of the chest cavity, between the lungs, the heart is about the size of your clenched fist. In shape, it bears some likeness to the Valentine symbol, but there the resemblance ends. In structure and function, it is about as tender, delicate, and romantic as a sledgehammer. Its thick muscular walls surround a cavity that is divided into right and left sides by a longitudinal muscular partition, called the septum. Each side of the heart is further sub-divided by a horizontal partition, which separates it into an upper thin-walled chamber, called the atrium (Latin; entrance chamber), which receives the blood, and a lower thick-walled pumping chamber, called a ventricle (Latin; small belly), which ejects the blood. The right side of the heart receives the used, oxygen-poor blood from the body and pumps it to the lungs, where it is re-oxygenated. From the lungs, the oxygen-rich blood returns to the left side of the heart. From here it is pumped through a large artery, called the aorta, to be distributed throughout the entire body. One-way valves between the atria and the ventricles prevent backflow into the atria when the ventricles are pumping. Similar one-way valves protect the mouths of the aorta and pulmonary artery, the blood vessel that carries blood from the right ventricle to the lungs (Figure 1).

Thus, the heart functions as a pump — but what a pump! Beating an average of 72 times per minute, day and night, it circulates the body's entire blood volume of five to six liters within a minute. In a 24-hour period, it pumps an amazing 2,192 gallons (8,300 liters), or over 792,510 gallons (3 million liters) a year!

The sequence of events carried out by the heart is referred to as the cardiac cycle. It is divided into a pumping phase, when it is delivering blood around the body (known as the phase of systole), and a relaxing phase, when it is receiving blood returning from the body and the lungs

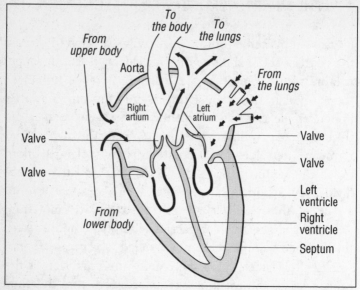

Figure 1: The Heart Pump
Four valves ensure that blood flows through the four chambers of the heart in one direction only.

(known as the phase of diastole) (Figure 2). When the heart is beating at its usual resting rate of 72 beats per minute, the systolic phase lasts about three-tenths of a second, and the diastolic phase five-tenths of a second. When the heart is beating much more quickly, for example during exercise, then both systolic and diastolic phases may be shortened by as much as 50%.

The environment of the planet Earth is unique (as far as we can tell to date). Its atmosphere consists of a mixture of gases containing 21% oxygen. Our bodies are designed to utilize that fact. If we are deprived of oxygen, the cells in our body begin to die, starting with the sensitive brain cells. Therefore the mechanism by which we extract oxygen from the air and utilize it is of paramount importance. This mechanism, known as the "oxygen transport system," works in the following manner: A series of feedback systems throughout the body keeps the brain constantly informed

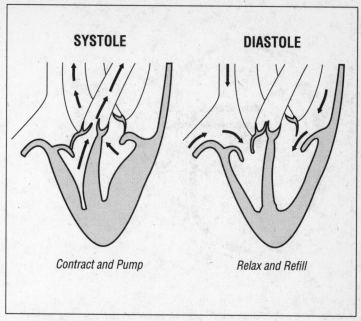

SYSTOLE   DIASTOLE

Contract and Pump   Relax and Refill

Figure 2: The Cardiac Cycle

of the level of oxygen in the bloodstream and the tissues. When the oxygen content falls below a critical level, the brain, acting through a relay of nerves, causes the diaphragm and the muscles between the ribs to contract. This increases the size of the chest cavity and creates a partial vacuum. Air is sucked into the expanding lungs and fills the tiny air sacs, or alveoli, of which there are literally millions in the lung tissue. Each alveolus is surrounded by a network of blood vessels called capillaries. When the air reaches the alveolus, it releases its oxygen, which then passes through the thin alveolar and capillary walls, into the bloodstream, where it combines with a protein in the red cell called hemoglobin (Figure 3). It is this combination, called oxyhemoglobin, that gives blood its bright red color.

The blood, now fully oxygenated, passes from the lungs through the pulmonary vein to the left atrium and then to the left ventricle. The left ventricle pumps the oxygenated

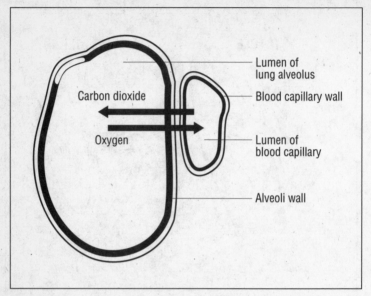

Figure 3: The Function of the Alveoli
Oxygen passes from air in the lung's alveoli to the blood in the capillary vessels through the two thin walls.

blood out through the aorta into the arteries, which branch into smaller arterioles, and then finally into the even smaller capillaries that course throughout all the cells of the muscles and organs. Once in the capillaries, the blood gives up its life-sustaining oxygen and receives in return the carbon dioxide and other waste products produced by the working cells. This oxygen-poor blood, now referred to as venous blood, is carried back through the veins to the right side of the heart where, as we have seen, it is pumped to the lungs. Once there it gives off its carbon dioxide, picks up its supply of oxygen, and the cycle starts again (Figure 4).

The heart, therefore, is the driving force of the oxygen transport system, the pump that must keep working day and night in order for us to survive. All very well, you say, but nowhere in this description is mention made of the method by which the heart obtains its own supply of oxygen-enriched blood. Since the explanation is vital to our

Figure 4: The Oxygen Transport System

Figure 5: The Heart's Blood Supply – The Coronary Arteries

understanding of heart disease, we will need to describe this in some detail.

The Blood Supply of the Heart: The Coronary Circulation

The heart receives its oxygen-rich blood supply through the left and right coronary (crown-like) arteries (Figure 5). They emerge from the root of the aorta and are the first of the many branches that arise from that large arterial trunk as it passes down through the chest and abdomen to the pelvis.

The left coronary artery, referred to as the *left main*, arises from the back wall of the aortic root and then quickly divides into two branches, the *left anterior descending artery* and the *circumflex artery*. The left anterior descending branch runs down the front of the heart to the tip, or apex, then curves underneath and ascends the back wall for a short distance. The circumflex branch encircles the left side of the heart to the back wall, giving off a branch that descends along the left margin of the heart. Thus between them the left anterior descending and circumflex arteries supply blood to the front wall of the heart, its left margin, and its apex. Interference with the flow of blood through either of these branches, but particularly the left anterior descending, would obviously jeopardize a major area of heart muscle. A blockage occurring higher up, in the left main artery, would be even more critical, since it would cut off the blood flow through both the circumflex and anterior descending branches.

The *right coronary artery* arises from the front of the aortic root, curves around the right side of the heart to cross the back wall (as the *transverse branch*), where it meets the end of the circumflex artery. It also sends a *posterior descending branch*, which descends the back wall to meet the terminal portion of the left anterior descending artery. The right coronary artery supplies blood to the right side and back wall of the heart.

Because the left main artery is so short and branches so quickly, we often refer to three rather than two coronary arteries, that is, the right, the left anterior descending, and the circumflex. All these branches feed a network of blood vessels that penetrate the muscular walls of the heart, subdividing into arterioles and then capillaries, providing a rich blood supply to the highly specialized heart cells.

This, then, is the coronary blood supply, a system that syphons off about one-twentieth of the blood that the heart pumps through the aorta every beat and redirects it back to nourish the heart itself. Considering its vital importance, the system should be problem free. Unfortunately, such is not the case. There are a number of flaws in the design, and they have a very definite bearing on the condition we now refer to as coronary heart disease.

The first problem has to do with the size of a coronary artery. Its inner diameter is not much larger than a drinking straw, and relatively minor encroachments on its inner wall can affect its ability to maintain a full flow of blood to the heart muscle. However, this would not matter so much if there were a rich, full, and plentiful network of inter-connecting arteries linking the three main branches. Unfortunately, this is not the case. The connections, or collaterals, as they are called, are relatively sparse and tend to come into play only when considerable narrowing has already occurred in the main stem branches.

Thus, the heart's blood supply can be threatened by anything that reduces the flow of blood through its already small-bore coronary vessels. The culprit is a condition known as atherosclerosis, the medical term for a patchy plaque-like accumulation of fat that occurs in the walls of blood vessels. Atherosclerosis can affect any of the small- or medium-sized arteries of the body, whether in the brain (where it can cause a stroke), or in the legs (where it can lead to gangrene), or in the coronary arteries (where it can cause a heart attack). We will consider the nature and causes of coronary atherosclerosis later. For now, let us examine its consequences: angina pectoris, acute myocardial infarction, and sudden cardiac death.

THE THREE COMPLICATIONS OF CORONARY ATHEROSCLEROSIS

Angina Pectoris

As the coronary artery becomes narrowed by the invasion of its inner channel, or lumen, by fatty patches, its ability to maintain a healthy supply of blood to the heart muscle gradually becomes impaired. For this reason, coronary heart disease is also referred to as ischaemic heart disease, ischaemia meaning "suppressing blood flow." In the early stages of coronary artery narrowing, or stenosis, there are no symptoms. This "silent" period is characteristic of the disease and may last for 20 to 30 years, depending on the aggressiveness of the atherosclerotic process. We know from examination of young American soldiers killed in Korea and Vietnam, and young Israeli accident victims, that coronary disease can begin as early as age 20.

Ultimately, blood flow through the coronary artery is so restricted that it cannot satisfy the demands of a fast-beating heart. Any number of things can cause the heart to beat faster: running, walking up a hill, climbing stairs, sexual intercourse, even high emotional stress such as an argument. When any working muscle is partially deprived of its blood supply, it develops a cramp-like pain. If you wrapped a tourniquet around your upper arm so as to cut off the blood supply, then clenched and unclenched your fist for a few minutes, you would soon develop severe pain in the muscles of your forearm. The pain would become increasingly worse until you were forced to stop making a fist. However, as soon as you released the tourniquet and allowed the blood to flow back into the forearm muscles, the pain would subside.

The heart muscle works the same way. Angina pectoris is no more than cramp-like pain originating from the blood-starved, or ischaemic, heart muscle. Classically it is felt in the middle of the chest behind the chest bone. Patients may liken it to "a rope tightening around my chest" or "something heavy sitting on my chest." The pain may radiate up to the neck and down one or both arms. Typically it lasts for minutes, rather than seconds or hours, and gradually subsides when the sufferer ceases whatever activity brought it on. As you can see, this description doesn't add much to that given by Heberden over 200 years ago, a testament to his acute clinical observational powers.

A common situation in which both the emotional and physical factors occur together is the all too familiar struggle through one of our modern overcrowded airports while carrying a heavy suitcase. As soon as our anginal victim slows down or stands still, the work load on the heart is reduced; the narrowed coronary arteries can now supply enough blood requirements to the heart, and the pain goes away. Although repeated attacks of angina are to be avoided, and doctors prescribe medication to prevent them, they are not the same as a heart attack. Indeed, anginal symptoms may persist for many years without ever leading to the second manifestation of coronary artery disease: an acute myocardial infarction, or heart attack. It is also important to understand that angina is due to a *temporary* shortage of blood to the heart muscle, which is corrected as the pain subsides, and does not cause any permanent damage to the heart.

Acute Myocardial Infarction (Heart Attack)

This term is used by pathologists and refers to the changes that occur in the heart muscle cells when they are permanently deprived of their blood supply. It represents a further stage in the progress of coronary atherosclerosis, although it often occurs in a patient who has never suffered anginal pain.

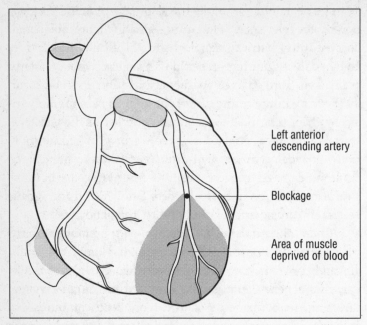

Left anterior
descending artery

Blockage

Area of muscle
deprived of blood

Figure 6: A Heart Attack

At this stage, the narrowed coronary artery becomes completely blocked, and the portion of heart muscle it supplies loses its blood supply and dies (Figure 6). The block may arise as the result of an atherosclerotic plaque enlarging so that eventually it completely fills the lumen. Or the surface of the plaque may crack, releasing a piece of its fatty substance, which is then carried downstream by the blood flow until it reaches a portion of the artery that is too narrow for it to penetrate. Finally, and this is the most frequent occurrence, a blood clot may form on the hard, cracked surface of plaque, critically increasing its size.

Death of heart muscle tissue is responsible for the classical symptoms of a heart attack. The patient complains of severe and continuous chest pain that, unlike angina, does not go away, even when he or she stops all activity and rests. There are all the signs of shock: sweating, pallor, slow pulse rate, and falling blood pressure. Within a few hours, the electrocardiogram tracing becomes abnormal because the electrical signals from the heart muscle are being modified by the presence of ischaemic tissue. There is also a rise in the blood level of various substances released by the breakdown of heart muscle tissue. These are known as enzymes; their diagnostic importance lies in the fact that they can often be detected by special laboratory tests prior to the appearance of changes in the electrocardiogram.

If the damage is severe, then the heart may stop beating ("cardiac arrest" or "ventricular fibrillation"), and the attack is fatal. If cardiac arrest occurs when the patient is already in hospital, then normal rhythmic beating may be restored by applying an external electrical current to the chest wall. This procedure is known as defibrillation. Obviously, there is a great advantage to having the patient in the intensive care unit; here the heart can be monitored continuously, and if cardiac arrest occurs, defibrillation can be carried out within seconds. Unfortunately, cardiac arrest is most likely in the first few hours of the attack, when decisions are still being made to call a doctor or arrange admission to hospital.

In recent years, a new form of treatment called thrombolytic therapy has been developed. In selected cases, and provided the patient is seen within six hours of the onset of the heart attack, anti-clotting substances are injected into the bloodstream to dissolve the clot in the blocked artery, restore normal blood flow, and reduce the extent of damage to the heart muscle. This will be discussed again later.

Occasionally, when the area of damage is large, the pumping action of the heart may be compromised, and the patient is referred to as being in congestive heart failure. With the advent in the 1980s of new and more powerful anti-failure medications, the outlook for patients who develop heart failure is greatly improved.

Sudden Cardiac Death

This third and most devastating manifestation of coronary artery disease is one of the major problems facing medical science today. It is defined as death occurring shortly after the onset of heart attack symptoms in a patient who is apparently healthy and who, up to that point, never had any symptoms of heart disease. When I tell you that sudden cardiac death accounts for about 50% of all heart attack deaths, you will get some idea of the magnitude of the problem. Autopsy invariably shows advanced coronary artery disease, even though previous symptoms have been absent.

CHD IN WOMEN

The three clinical complications of CHD — angina pectoris, heart attack, and sudden cardiac death — occur in women as in men. However, in women, angina is frequently the first symptom and it appears to follow a more benign course than in men. By this I mean that a woman may suffer from angina for many years, but not ultimately suffer a heart attack. In men the onset of angina frequently heralds a heart attack within a five-year period, unless suitable treatment is instituted. Although women are less likely than men to suffer a heart attack, when they do, it is more likely to be fatal. Of course, this apparent greater susceptibility to a fatal heart attack may not be so much due to gender as to age. Coronary atherosclerosis appears about ten years later in women than in men, and therefore those who progress to a heart attack are generally 10 to 15 years older than their male counterparts. They are thus more susceptible to complications, including chronic heart failure.

Sudden cardiac death, as distinct from a fatal heart attack, is a common cause of death in men. For some reason as yet unknown, women are much less likely to suffer from cardiac arrest and sudden death. In fact, the incidence in women is less than half of that in men.

STROKE

Atherosclerosis is the commonest cause of a stroke, a condition in which part of the brain is damaged as a result of being permanently deprived of its blood supply. Depending upon the extent and location of the brain injury, there is loss of speech, memory defect, behavioral disorders, and full or partial paralysis of either side of the body. Fortunately, with specialized rehabilitation, the outlook for full or partial recovery can be good.

Strokes are of two types, cerebral hemorrhages or cerebral infarctions. The former is due to rupture of an artery in the brain, with leakage of blood into the surrounding tissue. The cause of the break is weakness of the vessel wall, sometimes congenital, but usually as a result of atherosclerosis, combined with high blood pressure. In a cerebral, as in myocardial, infarction, the artery is blocked by a blood clot on the rough surface of an atherosclerotic patch. This type of stroke is also known as an ischaemic stroke.

The blockage may also originate in a clot located elsewhere in the body — the legs, lungs, or heart. A small piece of the clot can break off and migrate through the blood vessels to lodge in the brain. The migrating clot is called an embolus, and this type of stroke is called an embolic stroke.

Strokes are the third leading cause of death in the advanced countries. They are more common in those over the age of 55 and are one and a half times more prevalent in men than women. For some reason, the incidence of strokes has not escalated as dramatically during this century as that of heart attacks.

2. What Causes Atherosclerosis?

The specialist writing for the non-specialist reader is faced with the problem of presenting the subject as simply as possible without sacrificing fundamental accuracy. Obviously, too much attention to technical detail will make for tedious reading. On the other hand, oversimplification often leaves more questions unanswered than answered, or leads to confusion. The subject of heart disease and atherosclerosis is a case in point. In an attempt to educate the public, many health authorities have presented the disease in simplistic terms. Although I applaud their motivation, I cannot help but feel that this approach leads to problems of credibility down the line.

Almost everyone these days realizes that a heart attack is due to a blockage of a coronary artery. Many are even familiar with the term atherosclerosis. At this point, however, matters become oversimplified. Atherosclerosis is conceived as a blob of cholesterol sticking to the inner wall of the coronary artery. This blob is blamed on too much cholesterol in the blood, which, in turn, is blamed on eating foods high in cholesterol. Haven't we all been advised that too much cholesterol in our food or in our blood is dangerous? Mind you, many of us are not quite sure what cholesterol is, except that it is present in eggs and is presumably yellow in color. We also know from the labeling on food packages that any food that is "cholesterol-free" is safe to eat because it cannot give you heart disease.

If all of this is true, where does cigarette smoking enter the picture, or high blood pressure (doesn't that cause strokes)? What about diabetes, or stress, or family history or lack of exercise? And then again, if we are merely dealing with fatty blobs that are "furring-up the pipes," why can't we just inject something like a medical form of a Drano into the coronary artery that dissolves them? And what about those of us who have relatives or friends who consume prodigious amounts of fat, or smoke to excess, and yet live into their eighties or nineties? And finally, why do we continually read conflicting reports about the connection between heart disease and coffee, margarine, hard and soft water, and even viral infections? Sound familiar? With all these questions unanswered by the initial simplistic concept of coronary artery disease, is it small wonder that many healthy young adults are still sceptical about what they are told and remain reluctant to stop smoking, reduce the amount of fat in their diet, exercise regularly, etc.?

On the other hand, if we start with the atherosclerotic lesion itself, then examine the various theories that have been proposed to explain its presence in the coronary arteries, we might get a better understanding. I will do my best to make the following as simple and as accurate as the subject demands.

Remember the famous real estate dictum that the three most important features in a house are location, location, location. So it is with atherosclerosis. The first key to understanding the condition is to have a clear idea of where it occurs. It's a popular misconception that an artery resembles a simple pipe. On the contrary, the walls of the coronary artery, like those of all arteries, are composed of three layers, or coats (hence the Latin term *tunica*) (Figure 7).

The inner layer, called the *tunica intima*, is a single layer of flat smooth-surfaced cells, called endothelial cells. These are surrounded by a sleeve of elastic tissue. The tunica intima provides a silken surface over which the blood can flow smoothly and without interruption. It forms a resilient tube that can accommodate the pulsations caused by the heart's pumping action. Surrounding the tunica intima is the *tunica media*, or middle coat, the thickest of the three. It consists of smooth muscle fibers (so called because they are less complex in appearance than the coarser muscle fibers found elsewhere in the body), mixed with elastic fibers. This muscle layer can increase or reduce the flow of blood through the artery by constricting (vasoconstriction) or dilating (vasodilation) its diameter. Finally, there is the tough outer layer, the *tunica adventitia*, which consists of a combination of elastic and connective tissue. The adventitia supports the nerves that control vasoconstriction and vasodilation, as well as the tiny blood vessels that supply nutrition to the inner two walls. The inner channel itself is referred to as the lumen.

The mechanism by which the atherosclerotic lesion, or atheroma, involves these three walls is at the very heart (pardon the pun) of the debate over the cause of coronary heart disease. The term atheroma is a very old one. It is derived from two Greek words that, loosely translated, mean a tumor containing a porridge or gruel-like substance. In the past, it was used to refer to almost any tumor that contained a material of soft consistency. Only during the nineteenth century did it become associated specifically with the type of nodule or tumor that involves the walls of an artery. The most striking aspect of these nodules was that, when they were cut open, they were seen to contain a soft fatty material. Thus the term atheroma seemed appropriate. When it was further recognized that a later stage in the growth of the atheroma involved the development of harder scar-like tissue, and even calcium, the term atherosclerosis (fatty hardening) was coined.

Tunica intima (inner coat)
{
Endothelial cells
Connective tissue
Elastic tissue
}

Tunica media (middle coat)

Tunica adventitia (outer coat)

Figure 7: The Artery Wall with Its Three Coats

An atherosclerotic deposit advanced enough to reduce blood flow through the artery is seen by the naked eye as a raised, pearly-gray nodule that projects into the lumen of the artery. Under the microscope, we see that it also extends into the intima, through to the media and, in very advanced cases, even into the adventitial layer. The pearly-gray cap consists of scar-like fibrous tissue. Beneath the cap is a disorganized collection of smooth muscle cells that have migrated from the media into the intima, as well as a type of white blood cell known as a "scavenger" cell. Both scavenger and smooth muscle cells contain large amounts of a fatty material containing cholesterol, which is also seen in great quantities in the spaces between the cells. Additional contents of the deposit include flakes of calcium, as well as remnants of cells, which have lost a recognizable shape (Figure 8). In addition to invading the walls of the coronary artery, the nodules can spread sideways, involving long segments of the vessel.

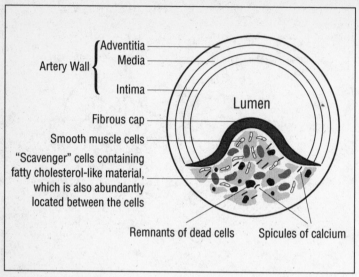

Figure 8: Atheroma
An atheroma with its contents. Note how it has invaded all three coats of the coronary artery wall and also projected into the artery's lumen, thereby obstructing blood flow.

So much for the lesion itself. What about the mechanism responsible for its presence? It is now generally accepted that the first stage in the development of atherosclerosis is injury to the artery's smooth endothelial lining. Early animal experiments in which the endothelial cells were intentionally damaged with an instrument passed into the coronary artery resulted in a number of responses. The first response involved a type of blood cell called a platelet. Platelets are tiny round cells, about half the size of a red blood cell, that circulate in the blood in large quantities. If there is a cut in the blood vessel wall, they prevent bleeding by gathering in clumps, sticking to the vessel wall, and forming a clot that plugs the hole. However, platelets are incapable of distinguishing between a break in the smooth cellular endothelial lining and a cut caused by an external object. As they clump around the injured endothelium, they not only cause a clot *inside* the artery, they release a substance

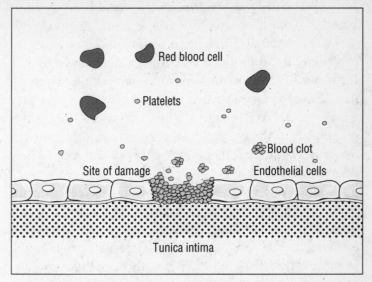

Figure 9: The Role of Platelets in the Formation of an Atheroma
**Blood platelet cells stick to damaged endothelial lining of artery,
clump together, and form a blood clot in an attempt to seal off
break in the vessel wall.**

that inflames the smooth muscle cells of the tunica media
(Figure 9). As a result, the inflamed smooth muscle cells
multiply, then migrate into the tunica intima, where they
then accumulate large quantities of a cholesterol-containing
fatty substance; they also form a scar-like tissue. In short,
experimental injury to the endothelium causes an atheroma.

The Causes of Atherosclerosis
The next question is clearly: what causes injury to the
endothelium? The three major risk factors that have been
linked consistently to heart disease are cigarette smoking,
high blood pressure (hypertension), and high blood cholesterol (hypercholesterolemia). How do these cause injury?
Cigarette smoke contains many chemicals with the capability
to damage the endothelial cells. Chronic high blood pressure
could also disrupt the endothelial layer by mechanical force

alone, particularly at the areas where the arteries bend or branch — which is precisely where most atherosclerotic deposits are found. It is not so obvious how an excess of cholesterol or fat in the blood damages the lining cells. On the other hand, substantial evidence has built up over the past 15 years suggesting that hypercholesterolemia *does* play a major causal role in coronary heart disease. Indeed, many proponents of the cholesterol theory maintain that it is the *only* cause. If the endothelial injury theory is correct, where does cholesterol fit in?

The answer has been sought in animal experiments. Although the evidence is not conclusive as yet, it seems that when blood cholesterol levels are high, the cholesterol particles are picked up by the scavenger white cells in the blood, and that these cells then pass through the apparently intact endothelium of the tunica intima to the elastic layer where they accumulate as a "fatty streak." The fatty streak grows in size, then ruptures through the overlying endothelial covering. The break in the endothelium then attracts platelets, which then initiate the inflammatory response that leads to an atheroma. Currently, this theory is a popular one, since it appears to fit the clinical facts.

There are those who reject the theory that high blood cholesterol initiates the formation of atheroma and who feel that damage to the endothelium, with resultant clumping of platelets and release of inflammatory "platelet factor," is the first step in the disease process. They point to the fact that the animals studied for the hypercholesterolemia theory are a specially bred strain of rabbit that suffers from a hereditary form of excessively high blood cholesterol similar to that seen in only a small proportion of humans. The human form of this genetic hypercholesterolemia is so virulent that it causes massive atherosclerosis and fatal heart attacks in very early adulthood. Can it be compared, they argue, with the moderately raised cholesterol levels seen in middle-aged adults, presumably as a result of a high-fat diet? Furthermore, the white scavenger cells do not have the ability to pick up cholesterol particles and carry them across the unbroken endothelial layer unless they are modified in some way. Such a modification — oxidation — has been shown to occur in the test tube, but has not as yet been demonstrated to take place in the living human subject.

You may think all this is merely splitting hairs. Not really. If high blood cholesterol is the sole cause of coronary heart disease, then all our efforts have to be concentrated on altering the dietary habits of the inhabitants of the developed world. If we accept only the platelet factor theory, then we have to concentrate on reducing hypertension, or eliminating chemicals or toxins that damage the endothelial lining or, alternatively, advocate the use of some substance, such as aspirin or fish oils, that may prevent the clumping of platelet cells. Nor is it beyond the bounds of possibility that there is more than one mechanism to explain atherosclerosis and coronary heart disease. For instance, high blood pressure, cigarette smoking, auto-immune disease, and even viral infection may result in physical damage to the endothelial cells. On the other hand, high blood cholesterol may lead to the release of substances from the endothelium that encourage fat to pass into the artery wall, without any apparent break in the endothelial lining.

We have to live with the knowledge we have at the moment. No one can now explain precisely and with absolute certainty the mechanism of atheroma formation at the cellular level. Nevertheless, we have gained considerable knowledge about heart disease, the factors associated with its development, and the techniques and strategies we can use to defeat it. We have achieved this knowledge by the use of the scientific method, which depends heavily upon the results of large-scale studies and trials involving hundreds of subjects over a period of months to years.

SCIENTIFIC STUDIES

In order to understand the studies and trials on which our knowledge is based, an understanding of the terminology is necessary.

Retrospective studies identify patients suffering from a disease and, through medical interviews and examinations, attempt to define which characteristics they have in common. For example, in the case of coronary disease, the common characteristic might be male gender or cigarette smoking; these are referred to as risk factors for coronary disease.

The predictive accuracy of risk factors can be tested by *prospective studies*. These identify healthy individuals who possess the risk factors, then follow them to see if they eventually develop coronary disease. Both types of studies make no attempt to affect the outcome; they are purely observational in nature. Probably the best known, and certainly the most often quoted prospective study in the field of coronary disease, is the U.S. Department of Health's Framingham Study, which started in 1949 and is still active.

In contrast, *clinical trials* test the effect on a disease of some form of intervention — either drug, diet, or even regular exercise. In order to avoid biasing the results by inadvertently preselecting a group of subjects who might respond favorably to the intervention, a process known as randomization is used. Candidates for the trial are randomly allocated, usually by computer, to either a treatment or non-treatment (control) group. In the case of a drug clinical trial, the control group is generally given a placebo, an inert, harmless substance identical in appearance to the drug. This corrects for the placebo effect, a well-known medical phenomenon in which some subjects experience a benefit from any form of treatment merely because they expect one. Since subjects do not know whether they are taking the active drug or the placebo, the trial is described as "blind."

When we come to evaluate the results of a clinical trial, we need to compare the occurrence of a predetermined measure, called the end-point, in the treated and the control groups; for instance, the occurrence of death from a heart attack. However, we have to be sure that any difference in end-points between the two groups is not due to chance. This is solved by subjecting the numbers to statistical significance testing. For a trial to show a statistically significant and conclusive result, the probability of any difference in end-point between the treated and the control subjects happening purely by chance alone must be 5% or less, expressed as p (probability) = 0.05. A probability of more than 5% (p = 0.06 or greater) means a non-significant or chance result. Obviously a probability of 1%, or one in a hundred (p = 0.01), or of 0.1%, one in a thousand (p = 0.001) confers upon the difference in end-point even greater statistical significance, and therefore makes it even more conclusive.

By now you should have a better understanding of coronary artery disease. We have reviewed its history, followed its disastrous path into the twentieth century, examined some theories as to its origins and causes, and outlined the methods we utilize to detect and deal with it in the community. The time has now come, to quote the Walrus, "To talk of many things"! Or, to be more precise, who gets heart disease, why, and what can we do about it?

3. Risk Factors

The studies that have been done over the past 40 years have identified certain characteristics and personal habits as increasing the risk of developing atherosclerosis. These can be divided into major and minor factors. The major can be subdivided into non-modifiable and modifiable.

Hypercholesterolemia and sedentary lifestyle will each be dealt with in separate chapters. This chapter will consider the two major non-modifiable risk factors — gender and heredity — then the remaining modifiable factors and the minor risk factors.

GENDER

Coronary artery disease is often referred to as a man's disease. This seems more than a little unfair. Many women suffer from angina; many have had a heart attack. In fact, the 3,000-year-old Egyptian mummy I mentioned earlier that was found to have a severe blockage of one of the coronary arteries was that of a 50-year-old woman. So why is coronary artery disease thought to be a man's problem?

MAJOR RISK FACTORS	
Non-modifiable	**Modifiable**
Gender	High blood cholesterol (hypercholesterolemia)
Heredity	Sedentary lifestyle
	High blood pressure (hypertension)
	Diabetes
	Smoking
	Environmental stress and personality
	Obesity
MINOR RISK FACTORS	
	Coffee
	Soft water
	Fibrinogen

Figure 10: Factors That May Increase the Risk of Heart Disease

The answer is to be found in the data obtained from the study of death rates from heart disease. If we examine the death rates from strokes in men and women over the period from 1900 to 1970, we will see that the ratio of male to female deaths does not change. However, from the 1920s on there was a steady increase in the number of males compared with females dying from heart attacks, the overall ratio increasing to as high as 3:1 or even greater (Figure 11). What's more, most of the men dying were between the ages of 35 and 65 (Figure 12). The current epidemic of heart disease thus commenced in the 1920s, and mostly attacks men in their middle years.

This evidence poses some questions. Why are men more susceptible, and why only since the 1920s? Does the female of the species have some gender-related factor that gives her an immunity from the epidemic? And, if the epidemic

Figure 11: Mortality According to Gender
Until the 1920s, the ratio of male to female deaths due to coronary heart disease was constant, then it began to rise steadily.
(Graph adapted from data published by Professor Terry Anderson at the International Symposium on Exercise and Heart Disease, Sponsored by the Toronto Rehabilitation Centre, 1979)

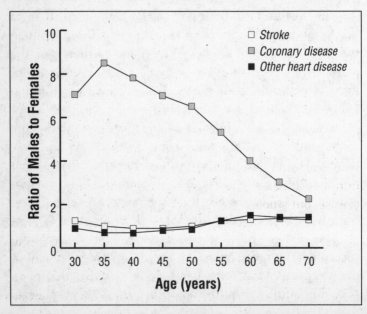

Figure 12: Ratio of Men to Women Dying of Coronary Heart Disease According to Age

is simply a twentieth-century phenomenon, why do women appear to have escaped scot-free? As women forsake their traditional role in the home and become more and more integrated into the hard-smoking, hard-driving, sedentary, fast-food set, will they come to equal men in their incidence of fatal heart attacks?

Female Hormone

Pathologically, the lower incidence of coronary deaths in women is explained by the finding that, when matched for age, women have considerably less extensive coronary atherosclerosis than men. The probable explanation is that the female hormone estradiol, a form of estrogen produced by the ovaries, protects women from the development of coronary atherosclerosis during the child-bearing years. After the menopause, estradiol production falls and is replaced by the less active estrogen, estrone, which is produced by non-ovarian tissue; the rate of atherosclerosis formation then increases. Attractive as this theory is, it is difficult to prove. Supportive evidence that the female hormone is protective is indirect and sometimes conflicting. For instance, in one study in which female hormone was given to post-heart attack males in order to prevent a recurrence, the result was the direct opposite: mortality from coronary disease was increased.

Women with a shorter lifetime exposure to estradiol — those who started menstruating in their late teens, or who reach menopause in their early forties — should, if our theory is accurate, have a higher incidence of heart disease, but studies have not shown this to be true.

In recent years, there has been an increasing tendency to prescribe estrogen therapy for women experiencing severe postmenopausal symptoms. The practice is not as yet universal. There is still debate as to possible effects, favorable or otherwise, on conditions such as female cancers, high blood pressure, or coronary heart disease. Physicians who do prescribe replacement hormones do so selectively, judging each patient individually and choosing for treatment those least likely to develop dangerous side effects.

Nevertheless, if we want to explore the question of female hormone and immunity from heart disease, it seems only reasonable to look at the incidence of heart disease in women receiving hormone replacement therapy. The majority of observational studies of these women show that postmenopausal estrogen users are at less risk for coronary disease. The most recent study, published in September 1991, comes from Dr. Stampfer and colleagues, of the Harvard Medical School, and involves 48,470 participants in the Nurses Health Study. The incidence of coronary events, fatal and non-fatal, in postmenopausal women taking estrogen was less than half that occurring in non-estrogen users over the ten-year period of observation. Other studies, however, continue to show that replacement hormones are also associated with a significant increase in the incidence of breast cancer, which could be coincidental, and a six-fold increase in the incidence of cancer of the uterus. However, since postmenopausal women have a 30% likelihood of dying from a heart attack, a 3% risk of dying from breast cancer, and only a 0.7% risk of dying from uterine cancer, the trade-off in benefit from reduced heart attack mortality might be considered worth it.

Some physicians feel that a conclusive answer can be obtained only by a prospective randomized clinical trial involving a large group of healthy menopausal women. They would be divided into those taking hormone and those taking a placebo. However, there are drawbacks. The cost would be prohibitive. Also, as previously mentioned, there is still debate as to the danger of prescribing estrogen to healthy menopausal women. It is difficult therefore to justify its use in a large population on the theoretical basis that it will prevent heart disease.

Assuming that female hormone does have a protective effect, we still have to explain how it works. We know that estrogens change the levels of the different types of cholesterol found in the blood. As you will learn later, cholesterol can occur in two different forms, low-density lipoprotein cholesterol, LDL-cholesterol, and high-density lipoprotein cholesterol, HDL-cholesterol. A high level of LDL-cholesterol is associated with coronary disease. In contrast, a high level of HDL-cholesterol protects from coronary disease. The effect of estrogens is to increase blood levels of HDL-cholesterol and at the same time decrease LDL-cholesterol levels. As a result, women in their reproductive years have higher levels of HDL-cholesterol than men. This differential diminishes after the menopause. Thus, it would seem that estrogen's effect on LDL- and HDL-cholesterol levels accounts for its protective effect. For the sake of completeness , however, I should add that careful analysis of the data shows that this accounts for only part of its beneficial effect. There are also data to suggest that premenopausal women have a degree of immunity from the two classical coronary risk factors of hypertension and diabetes. Also under investigation are the effects of estrogen on blood-clotting mechanisms.

The Pill
Another aspect of the female hormone puzzle concerns the birth control pill. During the 1980s, a number of reports linked heart disease with the use of the pill. Since the pill suppresses the function of the ovaries, using a combination of synthetic estrogen and its "antagonist," progestin, this result was not altogether unexpected. Once again there were confounding variables, such as a history of smoking, or the influence of aging. Smokers who were on the pill were reported to have as much as ten times the risk of a heart attack or stroke as non-smokers, with the risk even

higher in those over the age of 40. However, with time it became apparent that even more variables had to be taken into account. These included cholesterol levels prior to going on the pill, exercise habits, alcohol intake, the use of other medications, and so on.

Eventually, we have come to believe that it was the synthetic progestin in the pill that caused the increased incidence in heart attacks, but that this increase was relatively slight. Since then, newer pills have been devised in which the amount of progestin and estrogen are more evenly balanced. Recently, new progestins have been synthesized that do not harm the cardiovascular system. The most recent report from the Royal College of General Practitioners in the United Kingdom shows that birth control pills currently in use increase coronary risk only in those users who are heavy smokers. However, the heavy smokers were found to have 20 times the risk of CHD as non-smokers!

The Major Risk Factors and Gender

Even though younger women possess some gender-linked protective factor, we are still left with the unhappy statistic that coronary heart disease accounts for 373,000 deaths each year among American women. It is the third leading cause of death in women aged 35 to 39 years, the second in those aged 40 to 64 years, and first in women aged 65 and over. However, because of the greater male-to-female ratio of cardiac deaths in the age group 35 to 54, most of the research into the causes of coronary disease has involved men only. After all, if you want to learn as much as you can about a disease, it makes good sense to start by observing the group in which it is most prevalent. In short, you fish where there are the most fish. Or, as a famous bank robber replied when asked why he robbed banks, "Because that's where the money is."

But is it valid to assume that the conclusions gained from these studies on men also apply to women? In particular, do the same risk factors apply? With certain reservations, the answer would appear to be yes. What are these reservations?

Diabetes, when it is present, carries a two to three times greater coronary risk in women than in men. Furthermore, diabetic women have a higher prevalence of obesity, hypertension, and hypercholesterolemia than men.

Cigarette smoking is a particularly dangerous risk factor for women under the age of 50 years. In this age group, those who smoke more than 15 cigarettes a day are four and a half times more likely, and those who smoke more than 30 cigarettes a day, ten times more likely to suffer a heart attack than non-smokers. As in men, ex-smokers appear to be at little or no risk. As we have seen, smokers who are on the pill have as much as 20 times the risk as non-smokers on the pill.

Hypertension is less common in women under the age of 50 than in men; thereafter it is more common than in men. When it is present in women under 50 it seems to carry a greater risk than in men of the same age.

Generally speaking, premenopausal women have lower total cholesterol levels than men. Women who suffer from hypercholesterolemia, however, run the same risk as men. After the menopause, high total cholesterol levels do not correlate with coronary disease. The ratio of HDL-cholesterol to LDL-cholesterol is higher in women throughout their child-bearing years than in men, and as we have seen, this exerts a protective effect. However, after menopause, if or when HDL-cholesterol falls to low levels, the risk of coronary disease increases.

There have been conflicting reports as to the risk of obesity in women, although these disagreements may be explained by the relatively recent findings that the pattern of fat distribution is more relevant than the actual amount of excess fat. Women tend to put on weight around the hips, so that, even if they are obese, their hip measurement remains greater than their waist. Men tend to put on weight around the waist; all too often their belly protrudes well above the belt. It is the male pattern, whether in a man or a woman, that is associated with coronary disease.

Without getting into further discussion on the pros and cons of estrogen therapy, I should mention that premenopausal women who have had both ovaries surgically removed have a three-fold increased risk of developing coronary disease. If they are under the age of 35, they run a seven-fold increase.

There has been little investigation into the effects of such factors as family history, psychosocial interaction, or environmental stress on women. Nevertheless, from the Framingham and other studies, the following trends have emerged. A strong family history of coronary disease in young women carries an increased risk, but apparently this risk does not apply to women over 50. No difference has been observed in the incidence of heart disease between women who work outside the home and housewives. Women who have so-called Type A personalities have double the risk of their Type B counterparts (see page 71), although this may be related more to their smoking habits than to their personality. Even less is known about the effect of environmental stress on women compared with men. However, one intriguing research project has been carried out on a group of premenopausal macaque monkeys. The females of this species have a definite social status within their group and attempt to maintain or even improve that status (keeping up with or surpassing the Joneses, as it were). Over a ten-year period, batches of monkeys were exposed to stress by reducing their status and exchanging their dominant role for a more subdominant, submissive role. This change was achieved by putting them at the back of the line as they approached the water or food containers and depriving them of their rightful place to perch. All of the stressed females showed a marked drop in their HDL-cholesterol. Not only that, but they also developed severe coronary atherosclerosis. No such changes were observed in the non-stressed females. Further careful study revealed that the stressed females also showed an impairment of ovarian function, with the result that they had significantly lower levels of estrogen. This reduction in estrogen levels correlated closely with the fall in HDL-cholesterol and the appearance of severe coronary atherosclerosis. If we can extrapolate these findings to human females, then the implications are obvious. As more and more young women join the workforce, it is inevitable that an increased number will find themselves in stressful jobs — stock traders, air traffic controllers, firefighters, etc. Can we expect a female epidemic of coronary disease in the twenty-first century?

We know that more than 60% of all women who develop angina or suffer a heart attack have one or more of the known major risk factors. There is every reason to believe that, having identified these individuals, we should be able to take preventive measures that will be every bit as successful as in men. Unfortunately, we do not seem to have been as able to convince women of this as we might like to think. For instance, over the past 25 years smoking among men has declined by about 50%, whereas in female teenagers, it has increased. Obviously, when it comes to lung cancer and heart disease, we have been talking only to men. Contrary to the facts, women over 65 years continue to believe they are more likely to die from cancer than from a heart attack. We can only hope that future health promotion strategies will be designed with women in mind.

HEREDITY

As far as we know there is no specific gene for heart disease, although some families have a strong history of heart attacks. One likely explanation for this is the effect of family lifestyle.

Children afflicted with parents who smoke are likely to take up smoking. Parents with no interest in physical recreation are unlikely to have sports-minded offspring. A teenager accustomed in the home or at school to a diet of fast food or one heavy in animal fat and dairy products has probably acquired a taste for these items and may find it very difficult to change in adult life. There is strong evidence for this viewpoint. Studies show that the spouses of patients with heart disease frequently go on to develop heart disease themselves. Since the chances that both had a genetic predisposition to heart disease are very remote, the most convincing explanation is that they developed the same disease because they shared the same high-risk environment.

The Ni-Hon-San (Nippon-Honolulu-San Francisco) study examined the incidence of heart attack deaths in Japanese living in Japan and those who had emigrated to Honolulu and San Francisco. As is typical for their country, those living in Japan had few heart attack deaths. Those who went to live in Honolulu had twice the heart attack death rate and those in San Francisco four times. There was no reason to believe that the three groups were genetically different. However, the lifestyle adopted by those living in San Francisco was thoroughly North American, whereas those living in Honolulu retained some of their cultural identity, including their dietary habits. Similar observations have been made on Jews emigrating to Westernized Israel, where heart disease is common, from Yemen, where it is rare.

This is good news. We can prevent heart attacks by eliminating the modifiable risk factors. At the same time, it would be unfair not to consider the evidence of the influence of heredity. There may not be a "heart attack gene," but there is emerging proof that heredity does influence two of the major risk factors. For many years, it has been observed that high blood pressure tends to run in families, and a current theory has it that some of us inherit a tendency to develop this condition when exposed to certain environmental factors such as a diet high in salt or psychological stress. It should be noted, however, that the adverse environmental factors must be present in order for the genetic predisposition to take effect. In other words, both seed and soil must come together.

In recent years, the most intriguing and exciting discoveries have been made in the area of high blood cholesterol, or hypercholesterolemia. In 1986, a major breakthrough was made by Drs. Brown and Goldstein, two American scientists, which won for them the Nobel Prize. They established that the condition known as familial hypercholesterolemia was due to a genetic defect that led to the accumulation of high levels of LDL-cholesterol in the blood. Individuals with this condition invariably suffer a heart attack in their twenties or thirties, or in extreme cases in early childhood. It should be noted, however, that this disease exists in less than half of 1% of the population. But even here we are faced with the problem of seed and soil. In 1989, a unique study from the University of Utah traced the carriers of the gene for familial hypercholesterolemia through eight generations of a family that originated with a Mormon couple who were married in the 1790s. What emerged was a highly significant clue to our present-day coronary epidemic. Whereas those carriers living in the twentieth century either died from or developed manifestations of heart disease in their twenties or thirties, those who lived in the 1800s survived into their fifties, sixties, or even seventies. How could this be so? In the authors' words, "Male gene carriers born in this century tended to die at a younger age than male carriers of the same gene who were born in the nineteenth century . . . . It is likely that differences in diet or lifestyle may have affected disease severity in this family. The Utah pioneers were agrarian and physically active. Few members of this kindred living today have physically active occupations. Lifestyle and diet in the twentieth century gene carriers may account for the trend toward earlier death."

There is recent evidence of yet another form of genetic hypercholesterolemia. This form appears to be resistant to both diet and exercise, but may be controlled by LDL-cholesterol lowering medication. What seems to be emerging is that while some individuals inherit a susceptibility to atherosclerosis, they are probably balanced in the community by those at the other end of the spectrum who inherit a resistance to coronary disease, and that both groups make up only a small proportion of the population at large. Most of us are prone, not destined, to become victims of the so-called "good life" of the twentieth century.

HYPERTENSION (HIGH BLOOD PRESSURE)

What Is Blood Pressure?

Arterial blood pressure is expressed in two numbers, for example, 120/80 (stated as "one hundred and twenty over eighty"). The figures refer to millimeters of mercury (mm Hg). The first figure is the pressure in the arterial system when the heart is in the pumping phase of its cycle (systole) and is referred to as the systolic pressure. The second figure is the pressure when the heart is in the resting phase of its cycle (diastole) and is known as the diastolic pressure. The systolic pressure varies with the body's demand for oxygenated blood. For instance, during sleep when the muscles are relaxed, and all bodily functions are in the standby mode, the systolic pressure is low. During physical activity the working muscles burn oxygen at a faster rate and require an increased blood supply. The heart then steps up the speed and pressure with which it delivers blood into the arterial system. Thus the heart rate goes up, and the systolic pressure. During a bout of all-out maximal exercise, the systolic blood pressure can increase to as much as 250 mm Hg. This is considered a normal response. The diastolic pressure, on the other hand, represents the constant background resting pressure in the arterial system. Even during extreme exercise, it normally does not increase by more than 20 mm Hg, for example, from 80 mm Hg to 100 mm Hg. Our blood pressure is clearly not a fixed measurement, as many mistakenly believe; it constantly fluctuates.

If this is the case, how can your physician make a diagnosis of high blood pressure? Well, strictly speaking the diagnosis should read *"resting* high blood pressure." This measurement is made when a person is relaxed. The instrument used, called a sphygmomanometer, consists of an inflatable cuff attached to a pressure-measuring system, usually a glass column of mercury. The cuff is placed around the upper arm, just above the elbow. In this position, it lies over an artery, called the brachial artery, which runs down the inside of the arm crossing the front of the elbow crease. In fact, if you straighten your elbow and place your fingertips over the inner half of the crease, you will probably feel the brachial artery pulsating.

To take the blood pressure, the cuff is inflated until the pulsation of the artery at the elbow can no longer be felt. The pressure at which the pulse is obliterated is the systolic pressure. The examiner continues to inflate the cuff another 10 or 15 mm Hg above this point, and then, listening with the stethoscope over the area where the pulse was felt, slowly reduces the pressure. Nothing will be heard until the level of systolic pressure, at which point the pulse will reappear and will be heard through the stethoscope. The cuff continues to be slowly deflated until the sounds disappear; this point is the diastolic pressure.

Resting blood pressure can vary considerably in healthy individuals, with systolic readings ranging from 90 to 140 mm Hg and diastolic from 60 to 90 mm Hg. Anxiety is a well-known blood pressure stimulator, and even the very act of having it taken by a doctor can raise it by 20 to 30 mm Hg (the so-called "white coat" syndrome). Other factors that may affect blood pressure, particularly in sensitive individuals, are painful stimuli, extreme cold, or even the discomfort of a full bladder. The subject, therefore, should be comfortable and at ease in order to obtain an accurate reading.

Of course, the sphygmomanometer must be accurate. The inflatable cuff should be the correct size to wrap around the arm comfortably. This is particularly important in the very fat arm, where an ill-fitting cuff can cause an inaccurate reading. The reading is generally taken with the patient either lying down or sitting comfortably, with the arm supported at approximately the same level as the heart. Three readings are usually taken, and since the first two are often high due to anxiety, the lowest reading is recorded as being the most accurate.

In recent years, physicians have taken to teaching their patients how to take their own blood pressure at home. By looking at the measurements taken at various times during the day over a period of weeks, they can get some idea of what the true resting blood pressure is. Another recent innovation is the ambulatory sphygmomanometer, which uses miniaturized digital equipment to measure, record, and store pressure readings at regular intervals throughout the day. These can later be reproduced on a graph to show the daily fluctuations. Such devices are rather expensive and still have some teething problems, so are not in universal use. One early model made a soft but quite audible blowing noise as the cuff inflated and then slowly deflated. I recall giving one of these models to one of my patients to use over a 12-hour period. As it happened, he had to attend a protracted meeting of his board of directors the following day. Imagine his discomfort as on the hour, every hour, the directors were entertained by a short burst of soft but clearly audible snort-like sounds emanating from his person. Since they were too polite to enquire, and he too embarrassed to explain, the meeting must have been a memorable one.

Because diastolic pressure is less susceptible to transitory variations than systolic pressure, it is a better indicator of the day-to-day blood pressure level and is used frequently to define the presence or absence of hypertension. Why all this emphasis on the measurement of blood pressure? Because high blood pressure, sustained over a period of years, can have life-threatening consequences. It causes irreversible damage to the brain, heart, kidneys, blood vessels, and eyes. Unfortunately, it is not until the damage becomes obvious that symptoms appear and then it is often too late to do anything about it. Until then, high blood pressure causes no symptoms whatsoever, and its only sign is an elevated figure on the sphygmomanometer scale. It is now considered mandatory for everyone over the age of 30, and indeed even earlier for those with a family history of hypertension, to have their blood pressure checked annually.

What is normal blood pressure? A simple answer is the lower the better. It was thought that blood pressure increases with age, whence comes the outdated formula that a "normal" systolic pressure is "120 plus your age in years." Actually, only in urbanized industrialized societies does blood pressure increase with age. Primitive peoples living in their natural surroundings, such as certain groups of Australian Aborigines, the Inuit living in the Arctic, or the natives of New Guinea, have a low resting blood pressure throughout their adult years; it does not increase with age. In New Guinea and parts of South America where the incidence of stroke and hypertensive heart disease is extremely low, the diastolic blood pressure averages 60 mm Hg, approximately 20 points below the 80 mm Hg considered normal-average in our Western society.

RANGE (MM HG)	CATEGORY
Diastolic Pressure	
< 90	Normal BP
90-104	Mild hypertension
105-114	Moderate hypertension
> 115	Severe hypertension
Systolic Pressure, when diastolic BP is < 90	
< 140	Normal BP
140-159	Borderline isolated systolic hypertension
≥ 160	Isolated systolic hypertension
< Less than ≥ Equal or greater than > Greater than	

Figure 13: Classification of Blood Pressure Readings

Although elevated diastolic and systolic blood pressure usually go hand in hand, there is now strong evidence that an elevated systolic blood pressure on its own can be a powerful predictor of stroke and heart disease. Furthermore, whereas it used to be thought that an isolated high blood pressure found on a casual reading could be ignored, it now appears that this can be a warning of the future development of permanent hypertension, and therefore periodic re-checks should be arranged. Figure 13 gives the currently accepted levels for hypertension.

Consequences of Hypertension

The major ill effects of hypertension are two-fold: those directly due to the sustained pressure, and those due to associated coronary atherosclerosis. The constant high pressure in the arterial system throws an extra burden on the left ventricle of the heart, which compensates in the early stages by developing a thicker muscle wall, that is, it hypertrophies. Eventually, however, even the hypertrophied left ventricle is not up to the task, and it begins to weaken, dilate, and finally fail; it is unable to expel its entire contents with each beat, and blood begins to accumulate in the lungs. The patient notices increasing breathlessness, first on moderate then mild exertion, and finally even at rest. As the pressure backs up in the entire system, the right ventricle dilates, the water in the blood leaks out through the veins that return blood to the right side of the heart, and this excess fluid collects in the lower parts of the body, giving rise to swelling of the legs and feet. The patient is now in congestive heart failure. In addition to the direct effect on the heart, high pressures in the arteries to the brain, the kidneys, and the eyes can lead to strokes, kidney failure, and hemorrhages in the retina, respectively.

Hypertension is strongly associated with coronary atherosclerosis. Not only can it begin the atherosclerotic process by itself, it can also accelerate it in those who smoke or have high blood cholesterol. It is not clear how these effects occur. One explanation is that hypertension places an extra burden on the vessel wall and damages the endothelium. This theory is supported by the fact that atheromas frequently occur where the vessels branch or bend and are thus directly exposed to the full force of the blood flow.

People with hypertension are two to three times more likely to sustain a heart attack than those with normal blood pressure, and this risk is higher in those over 60. The heart attack is more likely to be fatal in these people. Sudden cardiac death is also three to four times more common.

Although our primary interest in hypertension is as a risk factor for coronary heart disease, it is clearly also a disease in itself, from which as many as 20% to 30% of North Americans suffer.

Types of Hypertension

Doctors distinguish between secondary hypertension and essential hypertension. In secondary hypertension, blood pressure is elevated because one of the organs of the body is diseased. The commonest cause is kidney disease. A diseased kidney releases a substance called renin into the bloodstream. Renin attempts to combat kidney failure by improving the organ's blood supply. It does this by increasing blood pressure, a scatter-gun approach at best. The kidney is helped only a little, whereas the cardiovascular system is seriously damaged. Secondary hypertension is relatively rare, comprising only about 5% of all cases of hypertension.

Essential hypertension occurs when there is no discernible causal disease; it is associated with 50% of all deaths in North America. It tends to run in families, with the child of a hypertensive parent more likely to develop it than one of a parent with normal blood pressure. If both parents are hypertensive, then the likelihood is even higher. Moreover, the more severely hypertensive the parents are, the more severe the hypertension in the offspring. Whether hypertension itself, or a susceptibility to developing hypertension in the presence of aggravating factors, is the inherited trait has not been established. What does seem to be certain is that there is a spectrum of environmental and acquired factors that, in certain individuals, enhance and accelerate the progress of the condition. These factors include age, body weight, diet, physical activity, and psychological stress.

Hypertension, Aging, and Obesity

In industrialized countries, people's blood pressure increases with aging, with about 50% of 65-year-olds being hypertensive. Since this is not seen in primitive societies, we can assume that hypertension in the elderly is not necessarily a feature of growing old, but is more likely a result of our modern lifestyle. One of the hallmarks of the affluent society is obesity. Surveys have shown that in the so-called advanced countries about one in five of us is overweight, and that one out of every three hypertensives is overweight. An Australian study estimated that in 60% of male hypertensives under the age of 45, the aggravating factor was obesity. When obese hypertensives lose weight, their blood pressure falls by about 2 mm Hg for every 2 pounds (1 kilogram) lost.

Hypertension and Diet

Various dietary constituents have been implicated in the development of hypertension. The one you are probably most familiar with is salt. There is a widespread impression that eating too much salt will lead to hypertension. This theory was based on early work that showed that populations with a very low salt intake had a low prevalence of hypertension. By the same token, communities whose population ingested large quantities of salt had a high prevalence of hypertension. Later studies, however, thoroughly examined the relationship between salt intake and blood pressure *within the same communities*. They did not find the same association.

A large international investigation known as the Intersalt Study has cast new light on the subject. Salt is a combination of sodium and chloride, and because sodium is believed to cause the problem, this study determined salt intake by measuring the amount of sodium excreted in the urine. The study, which involved 52 countries and some 10,000 subjects, found that in some of the primitive communities, low sodium excretion in the urine was associated with a low prevalence of hypertension. However, in the majority of communities studied, the relationship was not at all clear-cut.

What can we make of all of this? Well, if one in five of us is estimated to be hypertensive, then four out of five are not, even though we live in the same community and presumably have the same salt intake. The current thinking, then, is that hypertensives are sensitive to salt. There is no doubt that hypertensives who increase their salt intake will increase their blood pressure, whereas hypertensives who restrict salt intake will lower their blood pressure. Individuals with a personal or family history of hypertension should limit their salt intake to 0.15 ounces (4 grams) or less daily. This amount includes salt added during cooking and at the table, and also the hidden salt found in processed and fast foods. Canned meats, canned soups, hot dogs, potato chips, salad dressings, and bottled sauces are a few examples of foods loaded with salt. If in doubt, always read the label and avoid processed foods that contain added salt.

If there is a debate about salt intake and hypertension, there is very little about alcohol consumption. Since the 1970s, a considerable body of evidence has accumulated to show a direct relationship between drinking habits and hypertension. Fewer than two drinks a day apparently have no effect, but thereafter the risk increases steadily. Those who regularly have two to four drinks a day have twice the incidence of hypertension; more than four drinks have three times the incidence. (A drink is generally defined as one containing 0.5 ounces [15 milliliters] of absolute alcohol. This is approximately the amount in a 1½-ounce [approximately a 50-milliliter] shot of 80 proof liquor, or 3 ounces [approximately 90 milliliters] of 20% fortified wine such as port or sherry, or 5 ounces [approximately 150 milliliters] of a 12% table wine, or one 12-ounce [355-milliliter] can of 4.5% beer.) Incidentally, you can't save your daily allowance up and drink it all in one session, although you might want to divide your weekly allowance into two or three portions and indulge on two or three occasions in the week to give your liver some time to recover! Most physicians now advise even their mildly hypertensive patients to restrict their alcohol intake, and the more severe hypertensives to abstain completely. The good news is that the effect of alcohol on hypertension is quickly reversible, and is seen as early as two weeks after cutting back.

A number of other dietary elements are being investigated, but as yet there is insufficient data to draw firm conclusions. Primitive societies in which salt intake is low also frequently have a high potassium intake from a diet rich in fresh fruit and vegetables. In some studies, the blood pressure of hypertensives who were given potassium supplement dropped 5 to 10 mm Hg. The current Canadian guidelines for the treatment of hypertensives therefore recommend that hypertensives, in addition to reducing their salt intake, also increase their dietary potassium intake to the maximum.

Calcium, like potassium, might also help lower blood pressure. A number of large-scale nutritional studies have observed that hypertensives have a lower calcium intake. Experimental studies suggest that calcium supplements can decrease blood pressure in hypertensives. The recommended daily intake is 400–600 milligrams, and the most readily available source is milk, preferably in the form of skim milk, so as to avoid the saturated fat.

Whether a diet similar to that advocated for those with high blood cholesterol, that is, a diet low in saturated fat and high in polyunsaturated fat, can help hypertensives is still uncertain. Evidence in favor comes from the fact that vegetarians have a lower blood pressure than non-vegetarians. It seems unlikely that this is merely due to the lack of meat in their diet, but it could be the result of a low fat/high fiber content.

Hypertension and Stress
Although there is little direct evidence to associate hypertension with psychological stress, most physicians agree that many hypertensives are "race horse"-type people. They are often nervous and high strung and tend to react strongly

to situations they perceive as threatening. It has been suggested that, at least in the early stages, the hypertensive state results from the body's "fight or flight" reaction, which releases adrenaline-like hormones into the bloodstream. A side effect of these hormones is an increase in blood pressure. If this occurs frequently over a long period of time, the body becomes accustomed to this higher blood pressure level and allows it to become permanent. We will discuss this again later in the context of exercise and its ability to reduce stress.

A number of stress-relieving strategies such as hypnosis, meditation, biofeedback, and muscular relaxation are now commonly used to relieve stress, but unfortunately few have been thoroughly evaluated. Studies indicate that biofeedback can result in some improvement, but the long-term effect is small. Greater improvements have been seen with a combination of these techniques.

Hypertension Drug Trials

For many years, we have known that treating hypertension with drugs saves many lives by preventing strokes and congestive heart failure. We do not know, however, whether similar benefits would accrue to mild hypertensives, that is, those with a consistent diastolic reading of between 90 and 100 mm Hg and who, apart from this finding, are apparently perfectly healthy. In case you think that the problem is academic, consider the fact that 80% of all hypertensives fall into the "mild" category, which puts their numbers in the millions. If they were all to be treated by medication, the cost could be astronomical. Also, if the benefits of the treatment are slight or absent, large numbers of patients would be unnecessarily subjected to the potential danger of drug side effects.

In the 1970s, a series of large, multi-center, randomized, clinical trials was launched to answer this very question. In all, some 57,000 patients were studied, with the largest trials taking place in the United Kingdom (17,000 subjects), the United States (11,000 subjects), and Australia (3,000 subjects). All three major trials reported a reduction in strokes in one-third to one-half of the treated patients compared with the controls. However, whereas the benefit was obvious in those with diastolic pressures in excess of 100 mm Hg, the findings became a little less certain in those with lower readings. In the American study, there was a one-third reduction in strokes in those with diastolic pressures above 90 mm Hg. In both the Australian and British studies, however, there was no apparent benefit from drug therapy in those with a diastolic pressure below 100 mm Hg.

The other finding was more unexpected. Although fatal and non-fatal heart attacks were slightly reduced in the treated groups, this was not considered statistically significant, and certainly not as great as had been expected. A reasonable conclusion is that hypertension, while a major risk factor for a stroke, is less so for a heart attack. It also could be that hypertension needs to be associated with one of the other risk factors, such as hypercholesterolemia or smoking, to be a major risk for a heart attack. (Note that hypertensives who suffer from coronary disease frequently smoke, are obese, and have high blood cholesterol levels.)

Another explanation for this may lie in the drug treatment itself. In certain individuals, some of the medications used to reduce hypertension can have undesirable side effects, such as increasing cholesterol levels or accelerating the development of a diabetic condition. Therefore, individuals with diastolic pressures between 90 and 100 mm Hg should be checked every three to four months for any increase and, unless there are special circumstances (including hypercholesterolemia, diabetes, or a strong family history of heart disease), should be treated by drugs only if the diastolic pressure consistently exceeds 94 mm Hg (or 100 mm Hg, if you favor the more conservative British approach). In addition, vigorous non-pharmacological treatment is strongly recommended, including exercise, weight reduction, a low-fat, low-salt, high-potassium diet, abstinence from smoking, and restricted alcohol intake. Even when drug therapy is required, initial dosages should be low and should be supplemented with advice about a healthy lifestyle. We now have adequate evidence that even a modest reduction in pressure of 5 to 10 mm Hg achieved by non-pharmacological means can ensure that the patient is controlled on minimal drug dosages, or may even eventually be able to stop medication altogether.

DIABETES

The pancreas, a large gland situated in the abdominal cavity, secretes two hormones: glucagon and insulin. When blood sugar levels are low, glucagon stimulates the liver to release its stored glycogen into the blood in the form of glucose. When blood sugar levels are high, insulin facilitates the passage of glucose from the blood into the muscle cells, where it is burned for energy. In the condition known as diabetes, the pancreas is unable to secrete sufficient insulin, and glucose accumulates in the blood and spills out in the urine. The cells, deprived of the energy-rich fuel glucose, start to burn excessive amounts of fat or protein. This leads to the accumulation of toxic by-products in the blood, a condition that can cause coma and death. Diabetes was invariably fatal until the 1920s when two Toronto physicians, Drs. Banting and Best, isolated insulin from animal pancreas and successfully used it as an injectable replacement for human insulin.

Today, we recognize two main forms of diabetes, Type I and Type II. Type I is the classical form of the disease and the one most people are familiar with. Although it can appear at any age, it generally afflicts people under the age of 30. It is characterized by a total lack of insulin, requires full replacement therapy by injection, and is often referred to as insulin-dependent diabetes. Type II diabetes, or "late-onset" diabetes as it is also called, tends to develop in middle-aged or older individuals. The pancreas still secretes an adequate amount of insulin, but the cells are unable to utilize it, and in contrast to Type I, there are often higher than normal blood insulin levels. These patients become insensitive to their own insulin. Many Type II diabetics are obese, are hypertensive, and have high blood fat levels and low HDL-cholesterol (the "good" cholesterol) levels. In many, the diabetic condition may be reversed by weight reduction, a suitable diet, and an exercise program. In some, a hypoglycaemic (anti-high blood sugar) medication is also prescribed. Since insulin is not required, this condition is referred to as non-insulin-dependent diabetes.

It has been estimated that about 7% of Europeans and North Americans between the ages of 20 and 75 suffer from diabetes. Of these, however, about three-quarters have non-insulin-dependent diabetes, and in the affluent indus-trialized countries the numbers are growing rapidly. Approx-imately 20% of middle-aged and older individuals suffer from what is called glucose intolerance, a condition that precedes the development of non-insulin-dependent dia-betes. It is also referred to as chemical diabetes and can be detected by a glucose tolerance test. The blood glucose level is first measured after the person has fasted overnight. The patient then drinks a glucose solution, after which blood samples are taken every half hour for at least two hours and blood glucose levels measured. By the end of this time, the blood glucose, which has risen quickly after the drink, should have returned to resting levels. The extent to which it fails to do so is a measure of the patient's glucose intolerance (Figure 14).

Figure 14: Glucose Tolerance Test
After taking a sugar drink, blood sugar should rise within half an hour, then return to pre-drink level within one and a half to two hours. In diabetics, the initial rise is higher and the blood sugar level has not returned to normal after one and a half to two hours. This test can yield an abnormal result *before* the onset of diabetic symptoms, a condition known as chemical or latent diabetes.

Type II diabetics are two to three times more likely to develop coronary disease than non-diabetics. The premenopausal female diabetic loses her gender-linked protection and is four to six times more susceptible to heart disease. Even people with an abnormal glucose tolerance test, but who as yet do not have non-insulin-dependent diabetes, are at high risk. This risk persists, even when the influence of obesity, hypertension, and hypercholesterolemia, are factored out.

Despite the extensive research over the years into the effect of diabetes on fat and glucose metabolism, we are as yet unable to untangle all the mechanisms by which diabetes might be associated with atherosclerosis. Diabetics often have low levels of the protective HDL-cholesterol. They also have increased stickiness of platelet cells, which may contribute to excessive blood clotting. There is evidence that in diabetes an insulin-related substance may permit the passage of cholesterol particles across the endothelial lining of the coronary artery and therefore contribute to the development of an atheroma. However, to echo my old refrain, ignorance of the precise process or processes need not stop us from taking preventive action. Diabetics who are physically active, do not smoke, and have low cholesterol levels run a considerably reduced risk of disease.

CIGARETTE SMOKING

Few people are unaware of the connection between cigarette smoking and lung cancer. How many also realize that the smoker is three to four times more likely to experience a heart attack than the non-smoker, and that the attack is more likely to be fatal? The risk increases proportionally with the number of cigarettes smoked and is particularly high in those under the age of 50. The risk of sudden cardiac death increases more than ten-fold in men and five-fold in women who smoke.

The good news is that, at least in the developed world, the number of smokers has steadily declined since the 1970s. At the moment, about one in three North Americans is a smoker. It is estimated that by the year 2000, this figure will have dropped to one in five. The down side is that the figure would be even lower if it took into account only those who have and will in the future quit smoking. Unfortunately, since 1977 more and more people have started to smoke. According to the American Academy of Pediatrics, more than 3,000 children and teenagers in the United States start to smoke each day. Since the 1970s, there has been a sharp decline in the number of men in the 20-to-25-year age bracket who started the smoking habit. Over the same period, there has been a sharp increase in new women smokers in the same age bracket. If the trend continues, we can expect by the end of the century that more women than men will smoke. The British medical authorities have come up with the sobering statistic that of every thousand young adults who smoke, 250 will die from a smoking-related disease. In 1991, it was estimated that smoking will cost the U.S. economy more than $100 billion in health-care costs. The tobacco industry is now targeting the developing countries, and apparently with considerable success. Will these nations eventually have to face a problem of equal magnitude?

Tobacco smoke contains more than 2,000 known substances, including nicotine, carbon monoxide, nitrogen dioxide, benzine, formaldehyde, and hydrogen cyanide. Many of these compounds are capable of damaging the endothelial lining of the coronary arteries and thereby provoking atherosclerosis. Probably the two major harmful compounds are nicotine and carbon monoxide. The nicotine in cigarette smoke is highly addictive. It is released into the bloodstream within seven seconds of inhaling the smoke and almost immediately triggers the release of adrenaline and a related substance called noradrenaline. These two hormones, which are produced by the adrenals, two small glands just above the kidney, arouse and prepare the body for "fight or flight." As a result, blood pressure rises and heart rate goes up, increasing the heart muscle's requirements for oxygen. Unfortunately, however, this demand is thwarted by the action of the other substance in tobacco smoke, carbon monoxide, which is also the principal poisonous ingredient in car exhaust fumes. In large doses, carbon monoxide kills by displacing all the oxygen in the red blood cells. Actually, hemoglobin, the protein in the red cell that carries oxygen, *prefers* carbon monoxide and, given the choice, is 200 times more likely to pick it up than oxygen. You can see the paradox. Nicotine increases the heart muscle's oxygen requirements, and carbon monoxide makes sure that those requirements are not met.

If the coronary arteries are already narrowed and the blood supply to the heart limited as a result of athero-sclerosis, smoking makes matters worse. Anginal sufferers who smoke experience pain at a much lower level of exertion than non-smokers. Even in the absence of coronary athero-sclerosis, heavy smoking may cause heart attacks. There are reports of young heavy-smoking adults who have suffered a heart attack and yet on subsequent investigation are found to have normal coronary arteries. The mechanism is a shutdown of the coronary artery due to a spasm provoked by exposure to nicotine. In susceptible individuals, nicotine can cause life-threatening irregularities of the heartbeat. Sudden cardiac death is thereby probably another hazard for smokers. A number of investigators have also established that smokers have "sticky" blood and are liable to develop clots in their arteries, particularly the coronary vessels or the vessels in the leg. Finally, it has been noted that habitual smokers have lower levels of the protective HDL-cholesterol. Since a high HDL-cholesterol is felt to be one of the major mechanisms that protects young women from coronary disease, this might explain why women who smoke seem to have lost that protection.

It is extremely hard for most people to give up smoking. As an ex-smoker myself, I sympathize with anyone trying to quit. Experts in the field have said that in some ways addiction to cigarettes is as strong, if not stronger, than to heroin. The acute physical withdrawal symptoms may not be so severe, but apparently the craving is never quite extinguished. Many individuals who stopped smoking for 20 or even 30 years have started again after a few casual cigarettes. After 25 years of working with cardiac patients at the Toronto Rehabilitation Centre, we are now expe-riencing this phenomenon. Admittedly the numbers are small, but some people who were enrolled in our program in the late 1960s, and who stopped smoking after their heart attack, have started again after 20 years. To be honest, I have to say that if somebody were to offer me a perfectly safe cigarette now (and such a cigarette is nowhere in sight), even 25 years after quitting I would be tempted to start smoking again!

There is no safe alternative to quitting. Low-tar, low-nicotine filter cigarettes have been found to be just as dangerous as their predecessors, since habitual smokers will continue to get their boost of nicotine by taking deeper, more frequent puffs and smoking the cigarette right down to its filter. Pipe and cigar smokers are at slightly less risk than those who smoke cigarettes, but this is apparently not the case for former cigarette smokers. Having once learned to inhale from a cigarette, smokers invariably apply the same practice to a pipe or cigar.

How quickly after you quit can you expect to reduce your risk for a heart attack? Nicotine is quickly cleared from the body (which is why you experience early withdrawal symptoms). Carbon monoxide takes about 24 hours to clear, but by then its ill effects will have gone. One to two weeks after stopping, the risk starts to decrease, and a number of studies have demonstrated that it reaches almost the level of a non-smoker at the end of one year.

Danger to Non-smokers

In recent years, there has been increasing recognition of the dangers to non-smokers of sidestream smoke, that is, the smoke that escapes into the air from the burning end of the cigarette for all to inhale, smokers and non-smokers alike. In fact, this danger has been the major impetus for the banning of smoking in public places. Actually, sidestream smoke contains a higher concentration of nicotine, carbon monoxide, and other pollutants than exhaled (mainstream) smoke. Obviously, the danger to the non-smoker is greater in confined areas. A Scottish study, published in 1989, looked at the effect on a non-smoker living with a spouse who smoked. More than 15,000 men and women were followed up for an average of 11.5 years. The non-smoking spouses of smokers had two and a half times the incidence of lung cancer and twice the incidence of heart disease as the non-smoking spouses of non-smokers.

There has been a recent resurgence in the use of a very old form of tobacco, snuff. Oral snuff is now packed in small bags that are held between the gum and cheek. With the help of heavy promotion by the tobacco industry, and the example set by the "boys of summer," the baseball players, the use of oral snuff in the United States has increased 15-fold since 1970, largely in 17- to 19-year-old young men. Oral snuff, since it delivers nicotine to the bloodstream, albeit not so quickly as inhaled cigarette smoke, is nevertheless addictive and frequently leads to cigarette smoking itself. Apart from that, this form of tobacco causes cancer of the mouth, throat, and stomach. In 1990, Britain banned the sale of oral snuff, and similar bans are also in force in Israel, New Zealand, Hong Kong, Singapore, and Japan. How long will it take for North America to follow suit?

Years ago, more than I care to remember, when I first started talking to post-heart attack patients, I was often asked "How come my grandfather started to roll his own when he was 12 years old and smoked until he was 90, and he never had a heart attack or lung cancer?" In those days I would answer condescendingly, "Well, your grandfather isn't you, and you are not your grandfather. You are the one who has had the heart attack, and your grandfather was one in a million" — or words to that effect. In retrospect, I realize I probably antagonized the questioners and did nothing to convince them of the dangers of smoking. Now that I am older and, I hope, wiser, I would answer the question differently. I would admit that we don't have a full explanation for Grandfather's apparent immunity from heart disease (I can't speak for cancer), but the question is being researched fully and already there are some interesting data.

Take the situation in Japan. The incidence of coronary disease there is among the lowest in the world. On my first visit to that country, I was staggered to see how many men smoked. Subsequent visits confirmed this impression, and ultimately I was not surprised to learn that the Japanese consumption of cigarettes per capita is one of the highest in the world. This paradox is also apparent if we look at the data from a large international epidemiology study called the Seven Countries Study. This study looked at the risk factors for coronary disease in, as the name implies, seven different countries, one of which was Japan. Overall, while heavy smokers had a higher incidence of heart attacks than non-smokers, the relationship between smoking and heart attacks was relatively slight. However, if we pick out the countries with a high incidence of heart disease, smoking emerges as a risk factor, just as it has in other major studies carried out in the United States, the United Kingdom, Europe, and Australia, where heart disease is rampant.

The implication is that smoking often requires the presence of some other coronary risk factor, either known or unknown. Laboratory experimental evidence indicates that one of the major constituents of tobacco smoke, carbon monoxide, does not by itself cause any damage to the endothelial lining of the coronary artery, but that it will readily do so in the presence of high blood cholesterol levels. This connection would explain why smoking is strongly associated with increasing atherosclerosis in Western countries, where the average blood cholesterol levels are high, as opposed to Japan, where the average blood cholesterol levels are extremely low. Further evidence for the argument that smoking provokes coronary risk factors is found in the fact that hypertensives who smoke are five times more likely to go on to develop an extremely severe and often fatal form of the disease called malignant hypertension. Also, as we have seen, women smokers on the birth control pill have 20 times the risk of heart disease as non-smokers. Of course, none of this should be taken as a mandate for people without other risk factors to smoke. After all, the Japanese do suffer from lung cancer and have a very high incidence of stroke. Finally, if you live in the coronary-prone West, you might as well accept that the smoking habit puts you in double jeopardy.

Quitting Smoking

The acute symptoms of nicotine withdrawal last for about two weeks and, while not disabling, they are certainly not pleasant. They include irritability, insomnia, depression, and inability to concentrate. The more cigarettes smoked, the worse the symptoms. All strategies to stop smoking are designed to reduce the discomfort of nicotine withdrawal and then modify subsequent behavior so as to prevent a return to smoking.

It goes without saying that those people who are the most highly motivated to give up the habit are the most likely to succeed. One way to sharpen motivation is to spend a week or two writing down all the reasons to stop, to review the list daily, and then to inform family, relatives, and friends of the intention to stop — in short, to make it a big event.

Groups led by professional counsellors have about a 35% greater success rate over a 12-month follow-up period than those who tried to stop on their own. Once the program starts, the first aim is to reduce the effects of nicotine withdrawal. One way to do this is to use nicotine chewing gum, a prescription-only product. Used by motivated people in conjunction with group education and counselling, it has a reported success rate greater than 80%. In less-motivated individuals, or taken casually and without accompanying support, its results have not been quite so successful. Acupuncture was widely acclaimed for a time, but the initial enthusiasm for this approach seems to have abated. Hypnosis is still popular, and in the early days of the Toronto Rehabilitation Centre's cardiac program, we used it as an adjunct to exercise in postcoronary patients. It was reasonably successful in improving morale and self-confidence in certain patients, but the numbers were too small for us to judge its benefit in smoking cessation.

Some organized programs have a preparatory run-in, during which the subject is exposed to techniques that attempt to break the association between nicotine and a pleasurable sensation. Forcing oneself to smoke a number of cigarettes in rapid succession and rinsing the mouth with solutions that give a bad taste to the smoke are just two of the methods used. Again, the results have not been subjected to scientific trial, but patients who have attended these programs report some success. A gradual reduction in the daily consumption of cigarettes to soften the shock of the eventual cessation is another reasonable approach, and currently there is a small "computer" device on the market that signals when it is time for a smoke, the signals becoming less frequent over a two- to three-week period.

Once having stopped for two to four weeks, the individual faces the problem of relapse. During this stage the ex-smoker will inevitably begin to rationalize the need to start again. Weight gain is probably one of the most common reasons given, even though it rarely, if ever, reaches a level that constitutes a health hazard. An appropriate diet and a suitable exercise program can help avoid this consequence of stopping. A system of reward also helps. A good move is to put the money saved by not smoking in a separate bank account, and every six months spend some or all of it on some pleasurable luxury. Constantly reminding oneself of the health benefits of giving up can be a great incentive, as is the fact that food tastes better, clothes don't smell, and one is free from the never-ending fear of running out of cigarettes.

person makes up his or her mind ram of physical activity can be of workout releases into the blood- aaline, which can be a good substitute y improvement of fitness is tangible enefit, and the tendency to put on This approach worked well for me, my cardiac patients.

STRESS

ents referred to the Toronto Rehabil- iac program in the 1970s what they heart attack, six out of ten put stress at the top of their list. After attending for three months, they attached more importance to smoking, lack of exercise, and diet. Invariably, however, stress was still mentioned as an important factor. In the past three or four years, new patients have had a greater tendency to put diet on top, but stress is still considered important. Many people think that the stress of modern living is one of the main causes of our twentieth-century heart attack epidemic. Part of the reason we blame stress is that it is easier than blaming our own eating or smoking habits. Stress is something that our boss or the government or society has laid on us. It is beyond our control.

But although we all feel that stress must be a factor in coronary disease, few studies have addressed it. Part of the reason is that we do not have a satisfactory method to measure stress. In fact, there is no universally accepted definition of stress. The term was first popularized some 30 years ago by Dr. Hans Selye, who borrowed the word from physics. Dr. Selye used it to describe the body's responses to a variety of harmful physical stimuli, such as extreme cold or chronic sleep deprivation. These bodily responses are primitive and date back to a period early in our evolution when the environment was hostile but relatively simple. Faced with danger, primitive people usually had only two courses: stand and fight, or turn and run. Either way, excessive muscular activity was called for, and the body responded by releasing hormones (adrenaline and noradrenaline) into the bloodstream, which set the stage for action. These hormones increase the heart rate and blood pressure, thus ensuring a rapid delivery of oxygenated blood to the muscles. At the same time, they free up the stored fat and sugar from the fat depots and the liver, raising blood fat and blood sugar levels to make them readily available to the muscles for fuel. Breathing is quickened to augment oxygen uptake. Finally, and just in case the action results in cuts or bruises, the blood becomes "stickier" and will clot more easily to staunch any bleeding. The body is now like a tightly wound spring, straining to uncoil. This condition has been referred to as the "fight or flight" response (Figure 15). If physical action takes place, then the spring unwinds. Heart rate, blood pressure, blood levels of fat, sugar, and clotting substance all return to normal.

Let us apply this to modern life, where things are not so simple. Innumerable situations in our complex urban civilization pose a real or perceived threat to our peace of mind. Although the environment has changed, however, our response has not. It is still as primitive as ever. We are all familiar with the quickened heartbeat and breathing and the flushed face that accompany an argument or a feeling of panic. Rarely, however, is physical action an appropriate response. We cannot settle our day-to-day conflicts by fighting, or by running away. Nowadays, we rarely face physical dangers. Most of our problems are associated with personal finances, difficulties on the job, or interpersonal relations. Generally, these are solved with varying degrees of ease and form the background of normal living. This general level of tension is what Dr. Selye referred to as

Figure 15: Fight or Flight Response

eustress, or good stress. Without it, life would be dull, bland, and uninteresting. There is evidence that in the total absence of eustress, we would develop severe physical and psychological derangements. As a matter of fact, many of us crave a degree of potentially harmful physical stress. Why else do so many take part in dangerous sports such as mountaineering and climbing, automobile and motorcycle racing?

When does eustress become distress? Essentially, when we are faced with a threat to our well-being that we cannot solve. We are unable to cope. The spring is coiled, but there is no release. We are tense and anxious; our blood pressure, blood fat, and blood sugar levels are raised, and our blood is sticky and will clot easily. If this state of affairs persists in an individual who already suffers from narrowed atherosclerotic coronary arteries, then it requires no great stretch of the imagination to recognize the potential for a clot forming within one of those arteries, causing a heart attack.

This scenario is persuasive, and answers some of the apparent inconsistencies that arise from attributing the coronary epidemic entirely to a diet high in animal fat. For example, examination of the London Hospital's autopsy records for the period 1901 to 1952 reveals that over that period of time there had been no change in the extent of atherosclerosis in the coronary arteries. This evidence would suggest that our grandparents had just as much coronary disease as we have. On the other hand, from the 1920s on, there was a steady increase in the number of old scars detected in the heart muscle, a measure of the number of heart attacks that occurred during life. This finding would suggest that the change that occurred in the 1920s was not an increase in the extent of coronary atherosclerosis but some factor that increased intracoronary blood clotting. We shall look at this whole topic again when we deal with the relationship of physical activity to heart disease.

Establishing the mechanism by which stress can cause a heart attack still doesn't help us too much when it comes to identifying or quantifying it. What is stressful for one individual is pleasurable to another. Some of us delight in long hours and working to deadlines; others feel threatened and can cope only with the help of excessive alcohol, tobacco, or food. Contrary to popular opinion, many studies have been unable to find an increase in heart disease in high-level executives. Some 270,000 employees of the Bell Telephone Company were observed over a five-year period. Senior executives with heavy responsibility were actually found to have a lower incidence of heart attacks. Other studies in Sweden and Israel reached similar conclusions.

It is obviously very difficult to identify objectively a set of environmental circumstances everyone will find stressful. Nevertheless, efforts have been made to do just that. Probably one of the most widely used, the Social Readjustment Rating Scale, is based on the assumption that major life changes are themselves a source of stress because the adjustment they require imposes a psychological and physiological burden. If the adjustment period is lengthy, or a multiplicity of changes occur over a given period, usually one or two years, then the constant state of arousal ultimately breaks down the body's defenses and results in illness. The scale consists of 43 items, including "death of spouse," "divorce," "marital separation," "fired from work." While the authors of the scale found that retrospectively it correlated well with the incidence of heart attacks and sudden death, other investigators using prospective studies were unable to show any relationship between the scores and subsequent cardiovascular events. Another school of thought places less importance on the relatively infrequent major events in one's life and maintains that stress results from the accumulation of frequent daily irritants and events that force one through constant adjustment and adaptation. A list of common, minor irritants has been developed into the 117-item Hassle Scale, and initial work suggests that it might be a better predictor of stress-related illnesses than the major life-events approach.

Based on their studies, Drs. Mayer Friedman and Ray Rosenman have come up with a description of the coronary-prone personality. These aggressive achievers are ambitious and constantly attempt to accomplish more and more in less and less time. As soon as a goal is attained, they immediately set another, higher than the last. Characteristically, they are very time-conscious (woe betide you if you are late for an appointment with one), impatient (they rarely let the other person finish a sentence), speak in short explosive sentences, and are highly competitive. In short, they could be the role model for a highly successful businessperson. These individuals are classified as being personality Type A. In contrast, Type B personalities are described as less competitive, less time-conscious, more interested in cultural and artistic than business values, patient and relaxed. Type As, according to the theory, overreact to all challenges and are more susceptible to coronary disease.

This theory gained much support and a large following in the 1970s. Then in 1981 one of the first dissenting reports appeared. In a group of 189 heart attack survivors, X-rays of the coronary arteries (coronary angiography) failed to show any association between Type A personality and the extent or degree of coronary atherosclerosis. When these patients were followed up after discharge from the hospital, more fatal recurrent heart attacks occurred in Type Bs than in Type As. From then on, the case against the existence of a coronary-prone personality became even stronger. A complete review of all the data shows that whereas prior to 1977 the evidence was favorable, since then large well-designed studies have increasingly diminished the importance of Type A behavior.

Nevertheless, now that the initial fervor has passed, it may still be profitable to look more closely at the concept, since it still retains some tantalizingly attractive aspects. For instance, it has been suggested that a hostile attitude is the major component in a Type A personality that predicts future coronary events, and that current methods of screening are not sensitive enough to detect this hostility. Alternatively, if Type A behavior is harmful because it involves a constant readiness for "fight or flight," then measurement of heart rate, blood pressure, and blood levels of stress hormones, cholesterol, and sugar in response to a standard stressful task, such as solving a difficult mathematical problem in front of onlookers, would permit a more accurate and objective selection of the true hyperreactors than the presently used psychological interview and personality questionnaire.

Although the jury is still out, stress management has become one of the leading growth industries of our day. Books, audiovisual instruction kits, clinics, and counsellors abound. In the early days of the Toronto Rehabilitation Centre's cardiac program, we used hypnosis and later yoga to improve mood. Both methods had some success, but in our experience neither is as effective as a good exercise training program. In fact, for most of us, I would have to put exercise at the top of my list as the easiest, most readily available and successful method of coping with day-to-day stressful situations.

OBESITY

The word obese comes from the Latin *obesus*, meaning "that has eaten himself to fat." There couldn't be a better description of what has been identified as one of the most important public health problems for our times. The obese are prone to a long list of ailments, including heart disease, high blood pressure, Type II diabetes, gall bladder disease, cancer of the bowel and prostate in men, cancer of the breast and uterus in women, osteoarthritis of weight-bearing joints, bronchitis and asthma, accidents, etc.; the long list is frightening. Much of what we know about the dangers of being overweight has been gained from the massive amount of information gathered by the insurance industry. From their data, we have been able to formulate tables that relate body weight to height and also identify a "desirable" weight, above which there is an increased risk of illness and premature death. The most commonly used table in North America is the one drawn up by the Metropolitan Life Insurance Company, 1983 version. You can roughly calculate your ideal weight, if you are of medium frame, from the following: men — 106 pounds (48 kilograms) for the first 5 feet (1.5 meters), and 6 pounds (2.7 kilograms) for each additional inch (2.5 centimeters); women — 100 pounds (45 kilograms) for the first 5 feet (1.5 meters), and 5 pounds (2.3 kilograms) for each additional inch

(2.5 centimeters). If you are 20% above ideal weight, this is defined as being overweight; 30% above ideal is considered obese.

Lean Body Mass and Percentage Body Fat

You will note that the definition of the Latin word *obesus* used the word fat, and with good reason. When you step on the scales, you get a measurement of your overall body weight, which includes the weight of your fat mass *and* your non-fat mass. Your non-fat mass, referred to by scientists as your lean body mass, is the total weight of your muscle and bone tissue. Lean body mass usually varies with height, which explains why height and weight are linked in the Metropolitan Life tables. In healthy men, the fat mass is said to be 15% to 20% of the total body weight, and in healthy women 25% to 30% of the total. Excess weight is considered to be due entirely to fat mass. It is this excess fat mass that leads to the health problems associated with being overweight. Whereas the weight tables are a satisfactory guide for most of us, there are exceptions. For example, an ardent weight lifter or body builder will have excessive musculature and a disproportionately large lean mass. On the other hand, a very elderly person, in whom lack of any physical activity often leads to muscle wasting, will have disproportionately large fat mass.

If fat content is what we are interested in, why don't we measure it directly? The simple answer is that we do, but it's not as easy as it sounds. The most accurate method we have can be used only in a properly equipped exercise laboratory. It is known as underwater, or hydrostatic, weighing. First, you are weighed on standard scales on dry land. Then, sitting in a sling or suspended chair, you are totally submerged in a tank of water and weighed again. Since fat weighs less than water, you will weigh less submerged. The underwater weight is then subtracted from the dry weight and the result incorporated into a series of complex equations from which we derive a value for percentage of body fat.

An easier and more frequently used method is the measurement of skinfolds. The test is carried out by pinching a fold of skin and its underlying fat between the finger and thumb and measuring its thickness with a pair of specially designed calipers. This is done at several locations on the body. The measurements are generally combined in a mathematical equation that gives a predicted value for total body fat, although in some large-scale studies two or even one skinfold thickness have proved to be enough. This method is most frequently used by exercise physiologists, and in the hands of someone experienced in the use of the caliper and the correct choice of skinfold sites, it correlates closely with the results of underwater weighing.

You can obtain a reasonable estimate of your own fat layer by pinching a transverse fold of skin and fat over your abdomen, one inch (2.5 centimeters) below your navel. Ideally, this fold should be no more than half an inch (1 centimeter). The fat fold over the back of your upper arm, halfway between your shoulder and elbow, should be no more than one inch (2.5 centimeters) (one and a half inches or 3.5 centimeters in women).

Body Mass Index

The most universal method of measuring body fat is the Quatelet Index, or the Body Mass Index (BMI). This method has been adopted by Health and Welfare Canada and many other health professionals and government agencies throughout the world. The BMI is the figure obtained from dividing body weight by the height squared, that is, weight/height^2. Its purpose is to minimize the effect of height-related tissue (lean body mass). For ease of use, a "nomogram" (graph) has been developed that enables you to plot your BMI from your height and your weight and is shown on the next page (Figure 16).

A	B	C
HEIGHT (cm) (in)	**WEIGHT** (kg) (lb)	**BMI** (kg/m²)

Scale A (HEIGHT): 2.10, 6'10", 2.05, 6'8", 2.00, 6'6", 6'5", 1.95, 6'4", 1.90, 6'3", 6'2", 1.85, 6'1", 6'0", 1.80, 5'11", 5'10", 1.75, 5'9", 5'8", 1.70, 5'7", 5'6", 1.65, 5'5", 5'4", 1.60, 5'3", 5'2", 1.55, 5'1", 5'0"

Scale B (WEIGHT): 200, 440, 420, 400, 180, 380, 160, 360, 340, 320, 140, 310, 300, 130, 290, 280, 120, 270, 260, 110, 250, 240, 100, 230, 220, 210, 90, 200, 85, 190, 80, 180, 170, 75, 160, 70, 150, 65, 140, 60, 135, 130, 55, 125, 120, 50, 115, 110, 105, 45, 100, 95, 40, 90

Scale C (BMI): 50, 45, 40, 35, 30, 29, 28, 27, 26, 25, 24, 23, 22, 21, 20, 19, 18, 17

Figure 16: Body Mass Index (BMI)

To determine your body mass index: (1) Mark an x at your height on scale A; (2) Mark an x at your weight on scale B; (3) Use a ruler to extend a straight line drawn through your height and weight to intersect with scale C. Where the line meets scale C is your BMI.

A BMI in the range of 20-25 is generally healthy.

A BMI in the range of 25-27, though acceptable, should alert you to the possibility of developing health problems.

A BMI greater than 27 indicates the possibility of developing health problems, such as high blood pressure, diabetes, heart disease.

Note: BMI should not be used with children and those under 20 years, with adults over 65, with pregnant and lactating women, or with muscular individuals.

A BMI between 20 and 25 is considered to be desirable, since it is associated with the lowest risk of illness. A value of 25 to 30 is regarded as overweight. It represents a moderate degree of obesity and can be associated with some health risks. A BMI of 30 or higher is inevitably due to obesity and is associated with a higher death rate from the diseases listed above. Using this classification, figures from North America, Australia, the United Kingdom, and Europe show that about 35% of men and 25% of women fall in the category of moderately obese and a further 6% of men and 8% of women are markedly obese. It would seem that almost half the adult population of the industrialized world is too fat.

Body Fat Distribution

The diagnosis of obesity from height and body weight tables does not take into account the distribution of body fat, and there is new evidence to suggest that this factor is as important, if not more important, in identifying those at most risk from being overweight. Generally speaking, one can recognize two types of fat distribution in the obese. The first is the so-called android or male type, in which the fat is deposited on the trunk, particularly around the belly, increasing the girth around the waist. This is also referred to as truncal obesity. The second is the female, or gynoid type, where the excess fat is stored primarily around the hips and thighs (Figure 17).

In the mid-1980s, a series of intriguing reports from scientists in Gothenburg, Sweden, showed that truncal fat distribution, whether it occurred in women or men, could predict Type II diabetes, coronary disease, and stroke. Further evidence for these findings has accumulated since then, and it has become increasingly evident that the quantity of fat is not as important as where it is located. The truncal distribution can be easily determined by dividing hip measurement into waist measurement. A ratio exceeding 0.90

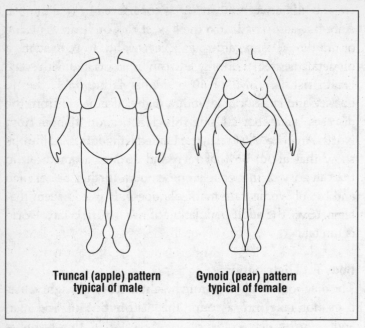

**Truncal (apple) pattern
typical of male**

**Gynoid (pear) pattern
typical of female**

Figure 17: Patterns of Obesity

in men and 0.80 in women indicates truncal obesity and increased risk. For instance, a man with a waist measurement of 46" (117 centimeters) and a hip measurement of 42" (107 centimeters) would have a ratio of 1.1 and would represent an obesity risk. A woman with a 26" (66-centimeter) waist and 36" (92-centimeter) hips would have a ratio of 0.7. If her hips remained at 36" (92 centimeters) but her waist increased to 32" (81 centimeters), the ratio would now exceed 0.8, and she would be at risk for obesity-related diseases.

Obesity and Heart Disease

There is a lot of evidence to show that obesity is a coronary risk factor for both men and women. A number of mechanisms could explain its adverse effects. Obese patients have a high incidence of hypertension, and the more obese they are the more severe the hypertension. When they reduce weight, their blood pressure starts to normalize. Type II diabetes and obesity often seem to go hand in hand. Whether or not they go on to develop a full-blown diabetic condition, obese patients frequently have an abnormal glucose tolerance test, which is in itself a coronary risk factor. Obesity is also associated with increased levels of blood cholesterol, but these increases are often small. Of greater significance is the more recent finding that obesity, as defined by the ratio of waist-to-hip measurement, is strongly related to low levels of HDL-cholesterol, the cholesterol associated with a reduced incidence of coronary disease. In fact, the term "Syndrome X" has been coined to describe a type of individual who has truncal obesity, glucose intolerance or true Type II diabetes, and a low HDL-cholesterol. Of course, all these features could be merely the result of many years of sedentary living and physical inactivity; nonetheless, combined they increase an individual's risk of disease.

Causes of Obesity

The children of obese parents often grow up to be obese themselves. Surveys show that when both parents are fat, three-quarters of their children will be obese; when both are thin, only 9% will be fat. This connection has led to the speculation that obesity is an inherited trait, and to the all-too-familiar argument between heredity and environment, or nature and nurture. Evidence in favor of heredity comes from studies of adopted children, who tend to take after their natural rather than their adoptive parents insofar as body build is concerned. By the same token, identical and non-identical twins strongly resemble one another in height, body weight, and fat distribution, regardless of whether they were raised together or apart.

A genetic factor does seem to contribute to obesity. Nevertheless, it is obvious that eating too much and exercising too little will make you fat whether you have inherited the tendency to become so or not. It may be easier to put on weight and more difficult to lose it if it is a family trait, but without the imbalance between high-calorie input and low-calorie burn, fat cannot accumulate.

The manner in which fat is stored also throws some light on the problem. The fat storage depots consist of collections of fat cells. We can increase the amount of fat in these depots in only two ways: the fat cells can increase in size (fat cell hypertrophy), or the fat cells can increase in number (fat cell proliferation). Proliferation is very active in the fetus during the last three months of pregnancy and the first year of life, after which it continues at a slower rate up until age ten or so, and then in spurts during growth periods of adolescence. There is generally little further increase during adulthood, although it can occur if the caloric intake is high and energy output low. Fat cell hypertrophy occurs in much the same manner, until by adulthood a maximum size has been reached. This size cannot be exceeded. One final point. *Once fat cells are added, they cannot be lost*. Therefore, weight reduction is achieved by *reduction in the size, not the number, of fat cells*. Because the number of cells remains the same, there is always the potential for them to pick up more fat, which explains why it is so easy to put on weight again after reducing.

Since cell proliferation is so active during early life, dietary and exercise habits adopted during this period have far-reaching consequences. Even the mother-to-be's pattern of weight gain during the final three months of pregnancy may be of considerable importance. For instance, we know that pregnant women who gain excessive weight during the final trimester frequently produce babies with a higher percentage body fat than those in whom the mother's weight gain was within desirable limits. Furthermore, if children are exposed to a sensible program of nutrition and regular physical activity, they are less likely to enter their adult years with an excess number of fat cells and to face a lifelong battle with obesity.

Surveys show that 80% of fat children grow up to be fat adults. As for adults, increase in body weight first results in the fat cells taking up more fat. Once they have taken on as much as their size will allow, additional fat can be stored only by manufacturing more fat cells. *This occurs when the degree of obesity exceeds 30% of the desirable weight.* Since weight reduction cannot be achieved by reducing the numbers of cells, the only alternative is shrinking the cells to a size less than that which has been genetically determined. This throws an extra burden on the body and makes weight reduction all the more difficult.

The Set Point Theory is yet another way of looking at the problem. According to this theory, everyone has a biological body weight that is compatible with good health. This weight is maintained by a center in the brain referred to as the "appestat." The appestat "sets" the individual's ideal body weight. When body weight strays too far from the set point, the appestat increases or decreases appetite and burns or conserves the body's store of fat. This theory explains why most of us maintain a fairly stable body weight, despite the day-to-day variation in the type and quantity of food we eat. There seems to be a genetic influence on an individual's biological set point since, as we have seen, there is often a familial tendency toward a heavy or light body build.

If the Set Point Theory is correct, however, why are some people obese? The answer lies in their lifestyle. We are not meant to be sedentary. Primitive people were constantly on the move, either hunting or foraging for food. Lacking this stimulus of physical action, the body senses that something is wrong, the appestat is set to a higher set point, and fat is conserved. The Set Point Theory thus explains why many weight-reduction programs don't work for the truly obese patient. Merely reducing caloric intake will only signal the body to conserve energy and protect its fat stores. If anything, the set point is raised even higher, as a form of protection against the next bout of what the

appestat perceives as a period of famine. Only by reprogramming the set point to its normal biological level can
weight be permanently reduced. This reprogramming is
achieved by a regimen of regular physical exercise combined
with a planned diet, the principles of which are a reduction
in fat and refined sugars, and an increase in complex
carbohydrates such as are found in whole grains, vegetables,
and fruit.

Regardless of the obesity theory, the plain fact remains
that the only way to maintain a desirable weight is to balance
your energy intake and your energy expenditure. A rough
guide to the number of calories you should be eating daily
is obtained from the following formula: take your desirable
weight in kilograms, allow 1 calorie per kilogram per hour
over a 24-hour period, and then add 30% to the result.
If you are very active, then you may add up to 60%. For
example, if your desirable weight is 70 kg, then:

70 kg × 1 × 24		=	1680
+ 30%		=	504
	Total	=	2184

If very active:			
70 kg × 1 × 24		=	1680
+ 60%		=	1008
	Total	=	2688

[Note: Divide your weight in pounds by 2.2 to obtain weight
in kilograms.]

Some experts who should know better have dismissed
exercise as an essential component of a weight maintenance
program. Their argument is that since there are 3,500
calories in a pound (500 grams) of fat, and since a 160-
pound (72-kilogram) person burns only 65 calories by
walking a mile (1.6 kilometers), then you would have to
walk 54 miles (87 kilometers) just to lose one pound (500
grams). This is an over-simplification. Apart from the effect
that a regular exercise program has on lowering your

set point, consider a situation in which you reduce your caloric intake by as little as 100 calories per day, and at the same time you walk one mile (1.6 kilometers) daily, to burn 65 calories. In 21 days, you will have lost one pound (500 grams) of body fat. If you walk two miles (three kilometers) a day you will lose one pound (500 grams) of fat in 15 days. Let's say you keep your daily 100 calorie restriction for one year, and walk two miles (three kilometers), five times weekly; at the end of the year you will have lost 20 pounds, or 9 kilograms, of fat. Furthermore, the fat will stay lost. Surely this is the sensible way to lose weight.

Look at it in reverse. It's a popular misconception that obesity is a problem of the middle-aged and elderly. Not so. As a matter of fact, in North America we gain most weight in our twenties and early thirties. Between the ages of 25 and 35, we put on about 7 to 10 pounds (3 to 5 kilograms). Five percent of that age group gain as much as 30 pounds (14 kilograms). The best way to avoid this is to exercise. Diet alone is not enough. Let us assume that a person becomes only slightly more sedentary over that period, just sufficient for his or her energy intake to exceed the energy expenditure by a mere 100 calories per week. That amounts to 104,000 calories over a 20-year period, which translates into an increase of 30 pounds, or 14 kilograms. So you see, even a relatively mild low-level exercise program can stave off the middle-age bulge. A brisk two- to three-mile (three- to five-kilometer) walk, five times a week, provided it is regular, will burn off excess calories, keep the fat bulge away, and prevent the loss of muscle bulk.

One often hears the plaintive cry, "I eat less than some of my skinny friends, and yet I still get fat." Numerous studies have shown that obese people are past masters at conserving energy. Scientists observing obese children in school and holiday camps have found that they are more sluggish in all physical activities. During field games, they move around as little as possible; during swimming practice, they rest much more frequently than their slim, active friends. As adults, they ride when they could walk, sit when they could stand, and even when sitting move around and fidget less than their thinner colleagues. The bulkier they get, the more difficult and uncomfortable it becomes for them to carry out any form of physical activity, and they are soon caught in a vicious circle. Even though they are eating very little, they are burning even less.

Weight-Reduction Strategies

For the truly obese, there are many commercial weight-reduction programs, each claiming to be more successful than the last. North Americans spend about $400 million annually trying to get slim — or about $160 for every pound lost (or $352 for every kilogram)! In general, however, the emphasis is placed entirely on reducing caloric intake. Some programs pay lip service to energy expenditure, offering brief and cursory advice to increase daily physical activities, but rarely is any effort made to draw up an exercise training program tailored to the client's needs. These diets can be categorized broadly into two groups: fad diets and semi-starvation diets.

The best-known fad diets advocate a low-carbohydrate, medium- to high-fat, high-protein combination. Initial weight loss may be dramatic, but this is largely due to water loss. The body stores carbohydrate in the muscles and the liver in the form of glycogen. The maximum glycogen storage capacity is 500 grams, or 1 pound. Each gram of glycogen is chemically bound to 3 grams of water, for a total of 1.5 kilograms or 3.5 pounds of water. With a shortage of carbohydrate in the diet, the reserve store of glycogen is quickly called upon, and as it is used it releases its water content to be excreted by the kidneys. Thus, the initial apparently easy loss of weight is not a loss of fat but of water and can be rapidly replaced. Only after the glycogen stores are depleted, and in the absence of a balanced diet, does the body start to use its fat stores. Not only that, but it also breaks down muscle tissue, with resultant muscle wasting, weakness, and severe fatigue. The substances released from the breakdown of fat and muscle tissue can also cause a series of side effects such as acetone-like breath, nausea, headaches, fatigue, and stomach upsets. Even after all this, studies have shown that the weight loss achieved is never permanent.

The semi-starvation diets are generally used only in cases of severe obesity, where body fat exceeds 40% to 50% of the total weight. These are usually carried out in a hospital, or under a doctor's supervision. Calories are drastically reduced in an attempt to force the body to burn its excess fat. Again, there is inevitable muscle wasting due to protein breakdown. Supplementing with vitamins and minerals, particularly potassium, is essential. Basic protein needs are satisfied by protein-containing food, or by use of a protein drink. Weight loss can be dramatic, up to 11 pounds (5 kilograms) in the first week, and 5 pounds (2 kilograms) every week thereafter. Constant blood checks are necessary in order to determine mineral loss, and supplemental minerals and vitamins are given accordingly. After about two to three months, the patient is gradually weaned on to a more balanced weight maintenance regimen. Initial results are good, but again these are rarely long-lasting. Some people have questioned the safety of this approach, especially when self-administered. Over the years, a number of deaths have occurred from cardiac complications during the diet.

In the final analysis, a balanced low-calorie diet is the most reasonable approach to weight reduction. The makeup of the diet should be approximately 50% carbohydrate, 30% fat (10% animal and 20% vegetable or fish), and 20% protein. It should typically allow for 1,200 calories a day, with an additional 30% to 60% depending on how active the patient is. The vitamin and mineral content should be adequate, and an accompanying physical training program specifically designed for the obese should always be prescribed. The aim should be to lose no more than 2 pounds (1 kilogram) a week.

Before leaving this topic, two words of caution. Although millions of North Americans are overly fat, there are many others, particularly young women, who strive for what they consider to be the perfect body. Even though they are a desirable weight, they perceive themselves to be fat and succumb to eating disorders such as anorexia nervosa and bulimia. It can only be hoped that a change in our cultural values and a stepped-up health education program will counteract this. Another cause for concern is the possible adverse consequences of losing and then gaining weight as a result of a series of unsuccessful dietary programs. This "yo-yo" effect has been the subject of a number of medical articles in recent years. Although not entirely conclusive, the data strongly suggest that this type of weight fluctuation is associated with an increase in fatal and non-fatal heart attacks.

OTHER RISK FACTORS

Coffee

Since the 1960s, there have been conflicting reports on the association between coffee consumption and coronary disease. The debate heated up when in 1983 a Norwegian study reported that people who drank nine cups or more of coffee daily showed a 15% increase in their blood cholesterol. Just when it began to look as if yet one more pleasure was to be denied us, an intriguing report from a group of scientists in the Netherlands appeared in the *New England Journal of Medicine* in 1989. These workers noted that the strongest evidence for the association between coffee consumption and serum cholesterol levels came from Scandinavia, where the coffee is made by boiling ground coffee beans and water in a saucepan and decanting the fluid into a cup. They carried out an experiment on 107 young adults who had normal serum cholesterol levels. Over a period of eight weeks, they were randomly assigned to one of three groups. Group one received four to six cups of boiled coffee a day, group two, four to six cups of filtered coffee daily, and group three did not receive any coffee. Those who had the boiled coffee increased their serum cholesterol levels by about 10%, while there was no change in the filtered-coffee group and the no-coffee group.

The following year, scientists from the Department of Human Nutrition in the Netherlands added further light to the subject. By centrifuging boiled coffee, they were able to separate a fat-containing substance they called "coffee fat." When this coffee fat was fed to a group of ten volunteers, cholesterol increased by an average of 25%. After the trial was terminated, cholesterol levels returned to normal. A further study by the same group showed that the coffee fat rises to the surface of boiled coffee, but in the drip method of brewing coffee, this fat is the last to drip from the funnel and does not pass through the filter paper. The lesson is that if you drink coffee, then you should use the filtered drip method.

Before leaving the topic, mention should be made of another study that demonstrated that people who switched from brewed coffee to decaffeinated coffee showed an increase in their LDL-cholesterol. No reason was given, and further reports on a larger number of subjects will be needed before firm conclusions can be drawn. The suggestion is that the bean used to make decaffeinated coffee is different from the regular bean. We are just beginning to recognize that there are a wide variety of substances in the coffee bean, many of which have not yet been identified, let alone been investigated for their possible side effects. Considerably more research is required in this area.

Soft Water

A number of epidemiological studies from around the world have noted that there is a higher incidence of death from heart disease in those areas where the water is soft. Unfortunately, no one has identified which specific component or components lacking in soft water may cause coronary disease. Since hard water flows over rocks rich in the mineral dolomite, it contains larger amounts of magnesium, calcium, selenium, and zinc. A low level of any of these substances in the tissues may, it is argued, affect the rhythm of the heart and, if the individual is already suffering from coronary atherosclerosis, predispose him or her to cardiac arrest. Conversely, soft water may contain increased amounts of manganese, lead, and cadmium, all of which have been reported to carry increased risk for coronary disease.

According to Dr. Andrew Schaper, a research worker for the United Kingdom Medical Research Council, the death rate from cardiovascular disease in Monroe County, Florida, was found to have dropped considerably after the water supply had been changed from a soft- to a hard-water source. Professor Terry Anderson of the University of British Columbia has verified that people living in soft-water areas have a lower magnesium content in their heart muscles than residents of hard-water areas. Since the hearts of people who have died from a heart attack are also found to have abnormally low concentrations of magnesium, he believes that water-borne magnesium exerts a protective effect. He also proffers the fascinating hypothesis that coronary heart disease is due to the critically low levels of magnesium in the highly refined Western diet, with the hard-water inhabitants receiving just enough to avoid a heart muscle deficiency state.

Despite what may appear to be impressive evidence, most workers in the field are quick to point out that the whole matter is still very much open to question. Certainly there are insufficient data to warrant altering the water supply of the nation, or to advocate that physicians prescribe oral calcium or magnesium for their heart patients.

Fibrinogen

In Chapter 2, I described how the formation of a blood clot on top of a coronary atherosclerotic deposit (coronary thrombosis) leads to a heart attack. The clotting mechanism is a complex one, involving the interaction of blood platelets and two protein particles in the blood called thrombin and fibrinogen. Once the platelets clump together, they start a series of reactions in which thrombin acts on the fibrinogen particles, joining them in long threads of fibrin. The fibrin threads form a meshwork that tangles and traps more platelets and red blood cells to form a firm clot. A number of prospective studies have shown that a high level of fibrinogen in the blood, like a high blood cholesterol level, is a major independent risk factor for a heart attack. This is particularly so in young men. However, while knowing that high fibrinogen may identify someone who is at risk for coronary disease sometime in the future, this knowledge does not help us in primary prevention. As far as we know at this time, there is no dietary plan or simple harmless drug that can lower fibrinogen levels and could justifiably be advocated for the population at large.

When I say that there is no public health strategy for lowering fibrinogen levels, I am speaking of the use of a specific anti-fibrinogen agent. However, there is evidence that high fibrinogen levels are directly associated with the other coronary risk factors, including cigarette smoking, high blood fat levels, obesity, hypertension, and glucose intolerance. Although direct experimental evidence is still lacking, it seems reasonable to suppose that any measures to eliminate these factors will also reduce fibrinogen levels.

We have covered a lot in this chapter, and before closing I think a short summary of the topics discussed is in order.

We have learned that the epidemic of coronary artery disease that commenced in the 1920s affects mostly middle-aged men. Women in their child-bearing years are relatively immune, but this immunity declines after the menopause. Medical science has established that those most likely to develop the disease have high blood cholesterol, are cigarette smokers, and often suffer from high blood pressure. Diabetes is strongly associated with coronary disease, especially in women. Obesity, particularly of the abdominal variety, is another risk factor. There seems to be little evidence that there is such a thing as a true coronary-prone personality, but there is a basis for believing that constant stress can ultimately lead to a heart attack. While excessive coffee consumption and living in a soft-water area have both been considered as contributing factors, their influence is small, and probably even then the mechanism is an indirect one that acts through some other agent as yet unknown. Heredity plays a strong role in only a very small proportion of patients with coronary disease; for the majority, environmental factors far outweigh the genetic aspect. Some authorities have identified abnormalities in blood-clotting mechanism as being important, but considerably more research in this area is required before it can be incorporated into a practical strategy for prevention.

It remains for us to discuss in more detail two other risk factors, hypercholesterolemia and sedentary lifestyle. Since, as Shakespeare said, "Delays have dangerous ends," let us proceed forthwith to those topics.

4. Cholesterol and Diet

If a creature from outer space were to make a tour of our supermarkets and grocery stores, it might conclude that one of our planet's major toxic substances was something called cholesterol. After all, package after package of food-stuffs proudly announce that their contents are "cholesterol free" or contain "no cholesterol." That same creature, were it to read a medical textbook, would be confused and mystified to learn that cholesterol is not a fat, but a combination of fat and alcohol, and that it is an essential constituent of all the cells of our body, particularly those that make up the tissues of our brain, spinal cord, and nerves. It is also a major ingredient of bile juice and helps to manufacture our body's supply of cortisone and sex hormones. Finally, it forms a protective layer in the skin, preventing the absorption of dangerous acids and solvents into the bloodstream as well as loss of body moisture into the surrounding air.

Without cholesterol, the human body could not survive. Cholesterol is widely distributed in nature and can be found in all animal products, particularly egg yolk and organ meats such as liver, kidney, and brain. We really don't need cholesterol in our diet, since our body can manufacture its own. This process takes place in the liver, which is capable of synthesizing up to six times more cholesterol daily than is found in the average Western diet.

If cholesterol is so vital to our health, how is it that products that have "no cholesterol" are widely advertised as being good for us? I explain this strange paradox to my patients by taking a look at how medical scientists sought to solve the puzzle of atherosclerosis.

Early Studies

As I pointed out previously, scientists first discovered that atherosclerotic deposits contained large quantities of cholesterol. Was is possible, they asked, that animals fed a diet high in cholesterol might develop atherosclerosis? The first answer to that question was published in 1908. It turned out that rabbits could develop severe atherosclerosis if they were given a diet rich in egg yolks, a prolific source of cholesterol. Of course, rabbits are not humans, and it was argued by many that, since they are vegetarians, the addition of any animal or animal product to their diet would be bound to cause some form of abnormality. Nevertheless, by the mid-1930s, as a result of these early experiments, atherosclerosis was thought to be a metabolic disease, caused by a defect in the manner in which the body either made or stored cholesterol. Finding a high level of cholesterol in the blood of people with coronary heart disease would, scientists felt, prove the theory.

For this reason, the principal investigators of the famous Framingham Study decided to include blood cholesterol, together with cigarette smoking and blood pressure, as the possible risk factors they wished to investigate. After all, it is fairly easy to measure blood cholesterol. The simple laboratory procedure involved had been used for years to diagnose various diseases of the liver, kidneys, and pancreas. Why not see if it had any value as a marker for the rapidly increasing disease, coronary atherosclerosis?

If the test had been around for so long, you may ask, why hadn't doctors already noticed that patients with high cholesterol levels were susceptible to subsequent heart attacks? The reason for the oversight lies in the way we determine normal and abnormal laboratory values. Blood cholesterol readings indicative of the non-coronary diseases just mentioned are either very low or very high. Thus, these levels became the reference points for abnormality. As for what is "normal," we also obtained these figures in the usual way — by measuring blood cholesterol in a large number of individuals, of all ages, in our community, and then taking as normal the *average* reading for the different age groups. Unfortunately, there was a potential for error in this method. Assuming that high blood cholesterol is a risk factor for coronary disease, then taking the average reading for a population in which the disease is rampant will give us a figure that might be average, but which certainly will not be "normal" or, to use a more accurate term, *optimal*. For instance, if you look at laboratory manuals printed as recently as the 1970s, you will find that for adults over the age of 30 years the normal range for blood cholesterol is 250 to 300 mg/dL (6.5 to 7.8 mmol/L).* The early Framingham results, however, showed that middle-aged men with blood cholesterol readings in that range were two to two and a half times more likely to suffer a heart attack in the future. What then was the level below which one was no longer at risk? After more than 30 years of study and observation, this level has recently been established as 200 mg/dL (5.2 mmol/L).

---

*Blood cholesterol levels are now expressed in the new Standard International (SI) units (mmol/L). However, because the older and larger units (mg/dL) are probably more meaningful to the public, they have been retained by the U.S. Public Health authorities for their National Cholesterol Education Program. Both methods of measurement will be quoted throughout this book.

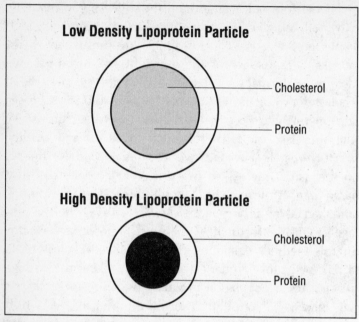

Figure 18: The "Good" (HDL) and the "Bad" (LDL) Lipoprotein

"Good" and "Bad" Cholesterol

Further refinements were to follow. To understand them, however, we have to make a small detour.

Cholesterol, like other fatty substances, does not dissolve in water. Yet it needs to pass from the liver, where it is made, or from the gut, from which it is absorbed, to and from the various tissues. The body's transport system is the bloodstream. Since blood is 80% water, fats will not dissolve in blood. The problem of how to transport these fats is solved by protein particles, called lipoproteins, which act as carriers of cholesterol and of the other fat molecules called triglycerides, of which we will speak more later. By making cholesterol soluble in water, the lipoproteins allow it to be transported in the bloodstream. Although very small, lipoproteins can be subdivided by their size and density into very low density (VLDL), low density (LDL), and high density (HDL) lipoproteins. An analogy for their size and weight might be, respectively, a soccer ball, a baseball, and a billiard ball. Triglycerides are carried almost exclusively by the "soccer ball" or VLDL particles. Cholesterol, on the other hand, can be carried by both the "baseball" LDL and the "billiard ball" HDL particles (Figure 18).

How does this relate to our story? In the early 1980s, the Framingham data clearly demonstrated that those who were at most risk for heart disease were those with high levels of LDL-cholesterol (LDL-C). It is still debated whether LDL-C rather than total cholesterol should be used as the first screening measurement to predict heart disease in the community. LDL-C is a better predictor, but at the moment it is harder to measure by means of laboratory tests.

In 1985, Dr. Michael Brown and Dr. Joseph Goldstein were awarded a Nobel Prize for their discovery of LDL-C receptors. You can think of these as sockets situated on the cell wall into which plug the LDL-C particles. The number of receptors are determined genetically, with one gene from each parent. When both genes are defective (homozygous hypercholesterolemia), there is a drastic reduction in the number of LDL-receptors. This occurs in about one in a million of the population. In these individuals, cholesterol levels range as high as 1,000 mg/dL (25.9 mmol/L), and fatal heart attacks generally occur in the teens. Where only one gene is defective (heterozygous hypercholesterolemia), a condition occurring in about 1 in 500 people, cholesterol levels exceed 300 mg/dL (7.8 mmol/L), and heart attacks usually occur when they are in their thirties or forties. In either form, even when blood cholesterol levels are optimal, there are insufficient receptors to accept a normal complement of LDL-C particles. As a result, the spare LDL-C particles circulate in the blood, becoming increasingly numerous and ready to contribute to the formation of an atheroma.

This discovery had implications not only for hypercholesterolemia, but also for the population as a whole, since it enabled us to see the problem of high blood cholesterol in terms of an imbalance between particles and receptors. Let us say that you possess a normal complement of LDL-C receptors, but eat a diet high in fat. You would then develop an excess of LDL-C particles in the blood. A proportion of these would soon occupy all the available receptors, leaving the remainder to be carried around aimlessly in the blood, unable, as it were, to find a parking space. Any breach or damage to the lining of the coronary artery would allow them to penetrate the artery wall and initiate the process of atherosclerosis formation. Since we currently do not know a way to increase our LDL-C receptors, our strategy has been to reduce the number of LDL-C particles, either by manipulating the diet, or if that doesn't work, by using drugs. Thus, even in familial hypercholesterolemia, manipulating the diet will help considerably by lowering LDL-C; drugs will lower it even further. From the Framingham data we have an optimal figure of 200 mg/dL (5.2 mmol/L) or less for total cholesterol. We know that approximately 60% to 70% of this cholesterol is normally transported in the blood by LDL particles. Thus a quick calculation gives us optimal value for LDL-C of 120 to 140 mg/dL (3.1 to 3.6 mmol/L). This is borne out by studies that showed that those with an LDL-C of 130 mg/dL (3.3 mmol/L) or less had the lowest incidence of coronary disease.

What about the smaller, heavier HDL-C particles? What role do they play? A most unusual one. In the mid-1970s, evidence began to accumulate suggesting that HDL particles are responsible for picking up any unwanted additional LDL-C and transporting it back to the liver, in the form of HDL-C, where it combines with the bile juice and is excreted in the bowel. This would imply that people with high levels of HDL-C could dispose of excess LDL-C particles and would therefore be less likely to develop coronary artery disease. This theory has been supported by epidemiological evidence, showing that there is an inverse relationship between HDL-C level and coronary disease; that is, the higher the HDL-C, the less the risk of a heart attack. Males before puberty and females before menopause have high HDL-C, after which the level drops and they both become susceptible to heart disease. Diabetics, cigarette smokers, and the obese also have low HDL-C. Whereas dietary measures can raise or lower LDL-C, HDL-C does not seem to be affected by these measures. It seems to respond favorably only to a regular exercise program and certain drugs. The optimal value for HDL-C is 35 mg/dL (0.9 mmol/L) or greater.

It now seems that one of the best measures of the level of cholesterol-related risk is the ratio of total cholesterol to HDL-cholesterol. This ratio is calculated by dividing total cholesterol by HDL-C; for example, total cholesterol 240 (6.1) ÷ HDL-C 60 (1.6) = 4:1. A ratio of 5:1 for men and 4.5:1 for women represents average risk. Our aim should be, therefore, to reduce this ratio between the two. It should be noted that while total cholesterol is a very reliable measurement in the hands of any general medical laboratory, and HDL-C is only slightly less so, LDL-C is not and has to be calculated from a formula that takes into account TC, HDL-C, and triglycerides. The suggested strategy for using these measurements to lower blood cholesterol in the population at large has been initiated by the United States National Cholesterol Education Program and, to a varying degree, has been adopted by most industrialized countries, including Canada and the United Kingdom. An outline of this approach will be presented later in the chapter.

To sum up, then, many animal, epidemiological, and experimental studies have demonstrated that elevated total blood cholesterol is a risk factor for coronary disease. Further information points to LDL-C as being the major culprit, with HDL-C exerting a protective effect. The optimal level for total cholesterol is recognized to be 200 mg/dL (5.2 mmol/L) or less, for LDL-C 130 mg/dL (3.4 mmol/L) or less, and for HDL-C 35 mg/dL (0.9 mmol/L) or greater.

Cholesterol and Diet: The Seven Countries Study

Nowadays few scientists would debate the fact that an elevated cholesterol is a strong risk marker for coronary disease. But this knowledge does not tell us how to correct the problem. To do that, we need to understand the link between blood cholesterol and diet. The first study to address this question started in the mid-1950s. Known as the Seven Countries Study, it was initiated by the American scientist Dr. Ancel Keys, and its findings are as valid today as they were when they were first published in 1970. Unlike the epidemiological studies referred to earlier in this chapter, which were all within-population, Ancel Keys's study was cross-population, involving approximately 10,000 healthy men between the ages of 40 and 59 from communities in Finland, the Netherlands, Italy, Yugoslavia, Greece, Japan, and the United States. When the study began, the subjects were checked for blood pressure, blood cholesterol, smoking habits, weight and percentage body fat, and resting electrocardiogram. They were then followed over a period of ten years for the occurrence of coronary disease. A fairly consistent relationship was found between blood cholesterol and heart disease, not only within the communities themselves, but dramatically so among the different countries. The country with the highest average cholesterol readings, Finland, had the highest incidence of coronary artery disease; in the country with the lowest average cholesterol, Japan, coronary disease was almost unknown. Strong correlations were also found in the United States, the Netherlands, and Italy. These findings confirmed, on an international basis, what had already been discovered in follow-up studies within single communities.

The next major contribution of the Seven Countries Study was that it detected the connection between a country's average cholesterol values and its dietary patterns. Careful inspection of dietary records and chemical analysis of food samples revealed that the inhabitants of countries where the customary diet was high in fatty foods, such as Finland and the United States, had average blood cholesterols well in excess of 250 mg/dL (6.5 mmol/L) and also suffered excessively from coronary disease. At the other end of the scale were the Japanese subjects who ate little or no fat, had an average blood cholesterol of 180 mg/dL (4.7 mmol/L), and suffered virtually no coronary disease. Of course, as with all multi-national studies, there is always the argument that some other cultural factor might be at work, apart from diet. This line of reasoning was directed particularly at the Japanese subjects. However, it was very satisfactorily countered by the Ni-Hon-San Study involving men of Japanese birth who had emigrated to other countries (see page 42).

THE CHEMISTRY OF FATS

The Seven Countries Study identified fat as the major dietary component responsible for increasing blood cholesterol to dangerous levels. However, this information led to further questions: What type of fat? And how much is too much? If we are to understand how Ancel Keys and his co-workers dealt with these problems, we have to take a quick look at the structure and chemistry of fat-containing foods.

The three major components of our daily diet are protein, carbohydrate, and fat. Protein is used for tissue building and repair, carbohydrate for fast muscle action, and fat for prolonged muscle action and long-term energy storage.

Pound for pound, fat provides more than twice the energy, or calories, of either of the other two foods. Its very simple chemical structure allows it to fold up easily for storage purposes. If we eat more protein or carbohydrate than we need, our bodies can convert them into fat, thus adding even more to our waistlines!

The fat molecule is called a triglyceride and consists of a combination of glycerol, a substance similar to glycerine, and three fatty acids (Figure 19). Ordinary everyday fat, whether it appears on our plate, bulges around our waist, or is carried around in our blood, appears in this form. Measurement of blood triglyceride levels is a routine procedure, usually carried out at the same time as blood cholesterol. Hypertriglyceridemia (that's right, medical terminology for high blood triglycerides) is usually associated with obesity and with diabetes. Whether it constitutes an independent risk factor for coronary disease at present remains uncertain, although recent evidence suggests that this might well be the case.

Figure 19: Triglyceride

The active portions of the triglyceride molecule are the fatty acids. As the muscles begin to use up their carbohydrate stores, they rely more and more on fatty acids as their long-term fuel source. As I said, a fatty acid is a very uncomplicated structure, consisting of a series of carbon atoms linked together in a chain, the monotony broken only by the attachment of hydrogen atoms and the occasional oxygen atom. Each carbon atom possesses four hooks, known chemically as bonds, which allow it to attach itself to other atoms. A fatty acid chain in which all the bonds are occupied is referred to as being saturated. Empty bonds fold up to form a double bond with their neighbor. Fatty acids with one double bond are referred to as mono-unsaturated, and those with two or more double bonds as polyunsaturated (Figure 20). The subdivision into saturated and unsaturated is of paramount importance.

How does all this chemistry relate to our foodstuffs? Our usual dietary sources of fat are animals, dairy products, grains, and fish. The triglycerides from all these contain varying mixtures of saturated, monounsaturated, and poly-unsaturated fatty acids. Animal fats contain a preponderance of saturated fatty acids. Vegetable and fish oils have a much higher proportion of monounsaturated and polyunsaturated fatty acids. However, three tropical vegetable oils — coconut, palm, and palm kernel — are exceptions. These contain large amounts of saturated fatty acids (Figure 21).

One further important point. As we all know, the present dietary trend is to substitute animal fats with vegetable oils — that is, to replace saturated with polyunsaturated fatty acids. This trend, however, poses a problem for the food industry. One can use liquid corn oil or safflower oil as a substitute for cooking lard, but what about a liquid substitute for butter? How would you like to pour corn oil margarine on your toast in the morning? The solution is something of a compromise. Food chemists have devised a method of partially saturating the unsaturated vegetable

$$-\overset{|}{\underset{|}{C}}-\overset{|}{\underset{|}{C}}-\overset{|}{\underset{|}{C}}-\overset{|}{\underset{|}{C}}-$$

A   A fatty acid, consisting of a chain of carbon atoms, each of which has four "hooks" or bonds.

$$H-\overset{H}{\underset{H}{C}}-\overset{H}{\underset{H}{C}}-\overset{H}{\underset{H}{C}}-\overset{H}{\underset{H}{C}}-H$$

B   A saturated fatty acid, in which all bonds are occupied.

$$\overset{H}{\underset{H}{C}}-\overset{}{\underset{H}{C}}=\overset{}{\underset{H}{C}}-\overset{H}{\underset{H}{C}}$$

C   A monounsaturated fatty acid, in which there is one double bond.

$$H-\overset{H}{\underset{H}{C}}-\overset{H}{\underset{H}{C}}-\overset{}{\underset{H}{C}}=\overset{}{\underset{H}{C}}-\overset{H}{\underset{H}{C}}-\overset{H}{\underset{H}{C}}-\overset{}{\underset{H}{C}}=\overset{}{\underset{H}{C}}-\overset{H}{\underset{H}{C}}$$

D   A polyunsaturated fatty acid, in which there are two or more double bonds.

Figure 20: Fatty Acids

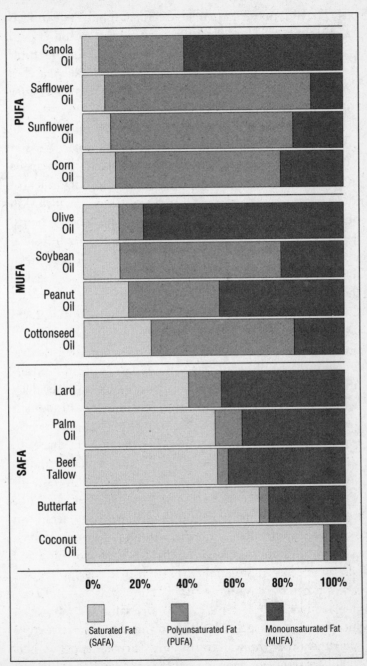

Figure 21: The Types of Fatty Acids Found in Common Dietary Fats

oils. They place the oil in a large tank and bubble hydrogen gas through it. This adds hydrogen atoms to the carbon chain. The process is known as hydrogenation, and the result is a vegetable oil with a higher melting point and a consistency closer to that of an animal fat. It is also easier to package and more appealing to use.

Hydrogenation is also used for another purpose. The empty spaces in the unsaturated fatty acid chain are just a little bit too available to any passing molecule that happens to be homeless at the time. The most commonly available molecule is oxygen; so, over a period of time, the inclusion of oxygen in the carbon chain causes the fatty acid to change its properties. It develops a rather unpleasant odor and taste. In other words, it becomes rancid. Obviously, if you attach hydrogen atoms to the spaces along the chain, you reduce the likelihood of rancidity. In short, if you want to prolong the shelf life of any foodstuff containing an unsaturated fat, you merely hydrogenate that fat.

Herein lies the problem. Hydrogenation defeats the whole purpose of eating unsaturated fats; since the unsaturated fatty acid is turned into a saturated fatty acid by hydrogenating it, you might as well eat animal fat. In addition to saturating the fatty acid chain, hydrogenation can also bend it from its normal shape (known as its cis shape) to a different, so-called trans shape. Some scientists, notably Professor Mary Enig, a biochemist at the University of Maryland, have consistently maintained that this change from cis to trans makes the hydrogenated fatty acid even more dangerous than a natural saturated fatty acid, such as occurs in butter, milk, or animal fat. Professor Enig and her supporters quote animal research that has shown that eating excessive amounts of trans fatty acids can not only increase blood cholesterol (as can any saturated fatty acid) but can also cause liver changes and alter the structure and function of the walls of the body's cells, reducing their ability to resist invasion by cancer-causing chemicals and interfering with their immunity response. Whereas our diet has always contained very low levels of naturally occurring trans fatty acids, over the past 20 to 30 years there has been a remarkable increase in our consumption of hydrogenated fats and oils, which contain trans fatty acids. Are we, by avoiding natural animal fats and substituting unnatural trans fats in our diet, merely swapping one evil for another? I bring this up not merely to be controversial, but because the topic emerges in the popular media from time to time, and since it is contrary to the current dietary advice, it confuses many patients and requires explanation.

Although, as we will see shortly, large amounts of hydrogenated fatty acids can increase cholesterol and elevate the fat content of the liver and kidneys in laboratory animals, they can only do so when the diet is also deficient in the naturally occurring polyunsaturated fatty acids, such as are found in the vegetable oils. Even then, long-term feeding studies have shown no change in the general health or longevity of animals given trans fatty acids. Neither is there any evidence to indicate that trans fatty acids play any role in the development of human cancer. Nevertheless, to ensure public safety, and recognizing the need for margarines and other vegetable oil products in the prevention of coronary disease, Health and Welfare Canada has recommended that all such products contain no more than 1% trans fatty acids and no less than 5% linoleic acid, the major polyunsaturated fatty acid.

How can you tell that the manufacturer has complied with this recommendation? To start with, it is rare for the label on the package to refer to either linoleic acid or trans fatty acid directly. Instead of linoleic acid, you will usually read "polyunsaturated fatty acid" (or PUFA); the margarine or shortening should contain at least 40% PUFA. Furthermore, it should contain no more than 25% natural saturated fatty acids. Finally, natural saturated fat *together with* hydrogenated vegetable oil should not exceed 40%. Many tub margarines and salad dressings nowadays contain little or no natural saturated fats, considerably less than 40% hydrogenated oils, and often more than 40% of polyunsaturated oils. However, if in doubt, read the label carefully. One brand of margarine, Becel, has avoided the problem of the trans fatty acids entirely by including a small amount (5%) of palm oil, which is made up largely of naturally occurring saturated fatty acids, in order to introduce a butter-like consistency to the product without having to resort to the hydrogenation process.

All in all, then, we cannot go wrong if we grasp the fact that hydrogenated vegetable oils behave like animal fats and so should be treated as such. However, there is no convincing scientific evidence that in the amounts found in the present North American or Western European diet they have any other harmful effect.

Dangerous Fats and Safe Fats

Now that we have defined our chemical terms, we can return to the work of Ancel Keys and his colleagues. The Seven Countries Study identified a fatty diet as an apparent cause of high blood cholesterol. This information, however, was not precise enough to be of practical value. Were all fats dangerous, or only certain types of fats? To answer this question, a series of feeding experiments was carried out. Volunteers agreed to follow a number of carefully prepared diets in the controlled environment of an institution. Differing quantities and types of fats were included, and blood cholesterol levels were measured regularly. In summary, the following very important findings emerged:

1. Medium-length-chain *saturated* fatty acids (with 14, 15, or 16 carbon atoms) raise blood cholesterol.
2. *Monounsaturated* fatty acids are neutral, neither raising nor lowering cholesterol levels.

3. *Polyunsaturated* fatty acids (the most important of which is linoleic acid) lower blood cholesterol.
4. Cholesterol itself, as contained in foods such as egg yolk and organ meats, tends to raise blood cholesterol, but not nearly so dramatically nor to the same extent as the medium-length-chain saturated fatty acids.
5. *Hydrogenated* polyunsaturated fatty acids raise cholesterol to the same degree as saturated fatty acids.

Ancel Keys's findings were so precise that he was able to predict what the blood cholesterol level would be if the diet were completely free from fat or cholesterol, and it turned out to be 164 mg/dL (4.2 mmol/L). From his experiments he then determined that if a specific quantity of saturated fatty acids raised blood cholesterol by a certain amount, then the equivalent amount of polyunsaturated fatty acids lowered it by half that amount. He expressed this in his now famous mathematical equation, the Keys Equation, which allows you to calculate your blood cholesterol, taking into account your total daily intake of calories, the percentage of calories from saturated and polyunsaturated fatty acids, and the cholesterol intake in milligrams. Blood cholesterol $= 164 + 1.3 \ (2 \times \text{SFA cals} - \text{PUFA cals}) + 1.5 \ \sqrt{1000 \times \text{chol (mg)} \div \text{daily total calories}}$. If mathematics is not your strong point, don't worry. The equation merely emphasizes the fact that saturated fatty acids are the prime constituents in the diet that raise blood cholesterol, and polyunsaturated fatty acids partially oppose their action. Total caloric intake is important, and dietary cholesterol plays a relatively minor role.

Let's pause for a moment and marshal the facts we have established so far. Starting with the early laboratory observations that atherosclerosis could be artificially induced in animals by feeding them a diet high in cholesterol and fat, we progressed to the studies, such as the Framingham Study, that noted a relationship between high blood cholesterol and the incidence of coronary artery disease. Ancel Keys, through the Seven Countries Study, demonstrated the link between blood cholesterol, dietary fat intake, and death from coronary heart disease. Feeding experiments then identified dietary saturated (animal) fat as the culprit, with polyunsaturated (vegetable and fish) oils exerting a partial protective effect.

There have been a number of additions to the original findings of Ancel Keys. None of these, mark you, overshadows the main thrust of his argument that the single most important dietary cause of hypercholesterolemia is an excess of saturated fat. However, let's now consider some of the more recent developments, including the role of dietary fiber, fish oils, and some new thoughts on olive oil.

Dietary Fiber

Dr. Dennis Burkitt first drew attention to the benefits of fiber in the diet while working as a medical missionary in Africa. He noted that disorders such as gallstones, bowel cancer, hypertension, and coronary heart disease were extremely rare among his African patients, and he came to the conclusion that their absence was due to the fact that the African diet contained a high amount of indigestible roughage, in the form of unmilled grains and cereals, or fiber. Over the past hundred years, this roughage has been gradually processed out of the Western diet. The effect of this lack of fiber in food is to reduce the bulk of the fecal stools and to increase the time of its passage through the intestine. Dr. Burkitt felt that the fiber in the intestine helped the body to excrete cholesterol through the bowel, and this contributed to the low blood cholesterol levels and consequent rarity of coronary artery disease.

Since Dr. Burkitt introduced his theory in the early 1970s, it has been widely accepted by the public and enthusiastically embraced by breakfast cereal manufacturers, who now vie with each other to produce a product with the highest fiber content. There was some disappointment, however, when controlled feeding studies carried out in hospital metabolic wards failed to show that dietary fiber had a cholesterol-lowering effect. There was good evidence that it benefited intestinal problems, but none that it could reduce the incidence of coronary heart disease significantly by altering cholesterol levels.

The matter remained in abeyance for a time, but then came to the fore again when it was realized that dietary fiber exists in a soluble and an insoluble form. Insoluble fiber is found largely in wheat, corn, and rice bran, as well as whole grains and nuts. When in the gut, it absorbs water and, because it is indigestible, cannot pass through the gut wall. Instead it forms a large bulky stool that is easily gripped by the muscular intestinal wall and quickly passes through the alimentary tract. The inclusion of insoluble fiber in the diet is considered beneficial in preventing some bowel diseases, possibly even bowel cancer.

Soluble fiber occurs as pectin in fruits such as apples, pears, oranges, grapefruit, and bananas; as glucan in oats and oat bran, bran cereals, whole grain breads, whole wheat spaghetti, peas, and beans; and as psyllium (sold commercially as the bulk laxative Metamucil), from the seed husk of the plantago, a grain grown in India. These fibers dissolve in water and form a gel in the gut. It was claimed that they could exert a cholesterol-lowering effect. Predictably, there was a surge of products on to the market containing soluble fiber, in particular oat bran.

One of the major proponents of oat bran as a cholesterol-lowerer is Dr. James Anderson of the University of Kentucky. He reported reductions in the order of 15% in cholesterol as a result of adding 50 grams (about a cupful) of oat bran to the diet of a group of hypercholesterolemic subjects. However, in 1990 a well-designed randomized study from the Harvard Medical School concluded that oat bran achieved its cholesterol-lowering effect not directly, but because it replaced saturated fat in the diet. After all, a large bowl of oat bran in the morning doesn't leave very much room for bacon and eggs. The investigators maintained that replacement of dietary saturated fat by *any* natural grain or carbohydrate would have the same effect, and that alone, without the addition of oat bran, would be equally effective in lowering cholesterol.

However, let us look at it in perspective. If oat bran works by helping you avoid saturated fat, why not use it? There is no evidence that it can do you any harm. And, as we have seen, there is every reason to believe that insoluble fiber prevents constipation and hemorrhoids, and possibly also diverticulitis and even bowel cancer. In any event, the story isn't quite over yet. In 1991, a group of investigators from the Chicago Center for Clinical Research published the results of their study on the hypocholesterolemic effects of glucan in oat bran. Oat bran, although similar calorically to oatmeal, contains more of the soluble fiber glucan than oatmeal. The researchers took a group of 156 adults who already had high levels of blood cholesterol and also suffered from multiple risk factors for heart disease. They were randomized into three groups. For six weeks, one received supplements of oatmeal, the second oat bran, and the third a placebo. In addition, all were placed on the American Heart Association Diet, with the same number of calories and the same amount of saturated fat. At the end of the experiment, the placebo group, as might be expected, had no change in cholesterol levels. Supplementation with 2 ounces (57 grams) of oat bran resulted in a 16% drop in LDL-cholesterol, whereas 3 ounces (85 grams) of oatmeal was required to produce an 11.5% reduction. Finally, after a further six weeks' "wash out" during which supplementation was withheld, cholesterol levels returned to their pre-experiment values. The implication here is that the soluble fiber does indeed lower blood cholesterol and is a valuable supplement to those high-risk individuals who are following the American Heart Association Low-Fat Diet. Of course, further randomized trials are necessary in order to see what the long-term effect of oat bran supplementation would be.

Psyllium, taken in the form of Metamucil in doses of one rounded teaspoon in a glass of water once or twice a day, has also been shown to reduce cholesterol by approximately 5%. Higher doses may have a greater effect, but recently there have been reports of individuals developing severe allergic reactions to Metamucil. Although such cases are rare, care should be taken if using it for the first time.

The more general complaints of first-time users of any of the dietary fibers are gas and bloating. These can usually be avoided if you increase your fiber intake gradually. Under normal circumstances you probably don't require more than 2 ounces (57 grams) daily.

Currently, North Americans consume one-third to one-half an ounce (about 10 to 14 grams) of fiber a day. The American Dietary Association and the National Cancer Institute recommend 1 ounce (28 grams) of fiber a day, one-third of which should be soluble fiber.

Before leaving the topic, I should emphasize that the overall effect of dietary fiber on blood cholesterol is relatively modest. *Hypercholesterolemia is primarily associated with eating too much saturated fat, not from eating too little fiber.* The place for fiber is as a supplement to a low-fat diet. Remember too that hydrogenated vegetable oil acts as a saturated fat, whether or not it is combined with fiber. There is little point in buying commercially prepared oat bran muffins that include in their list of ingredients a hefty quantity of fully hydrogenated oil.

Fish Oils

During the early 1970s, Danish medical scientist Dr. Jorn Dyerberg investigated reports that Greenland Inuit had only about one-tenth the incidence of heart attacks that their

Danish counterparts had. Since Inuit people who had migrated to Denmark lost this immunity, the protective factor seemed more likely environmental than genetic. A careful study of the Inuit lifestyle identified their diet as containing the protective factor. In Greenland, the Inuit diet is largely composed of cold water ocean fish. These creatures contain an oil that is high in two polyunsaturated fatty acids, eicosapentaenoic acid and docosahexaenoic acid. They are also referred to as the Omega-3 fatty acids. Over the past 15 years, considerable research has been carried out on the Omega-3s. They appear to benefit the cardiovascular system not so much by altering blood fats (although they do lower blood triglyceride levels), but rather by reducing the tendency of blood to clot within the coronary arteries. This benefit would explain the reduced incidence of heart attack deaths not only in the Greenland Inuit, but also the Japanese, whose diet contains an average per capita consumption of 3.5 ounces (100 grams) of fish per day.

For most of us, the best way to increase our intake of Omega-3 fatty acids is to include a meal of cold water fish in our diet two or more times weekly. In fact, eating fish even once or twice a week may protect us from coronary disease, as a 20-year follow-up of the inhabitants of the small town of Zutphen in the Netherlands has shown. Among those who averaged as little as 7 ounces (200 grams) of fish weekly there were two and a half times fewer deaths from heart attacks than among non-fish eaters. The major sources of Omega-3 are anchovies, herring, mackerel, salmon, sardines, tuna, and white fish. As a rule, the darker the flesh of the fish, the higher the Omega-3 content. The canned variety is quite suitable, since the fish oil is in the meat. However, don't be fooled by the oil in which it is canned. In the case of sardines and tuna, this is often a vegetable, not an Omega-3, oil.

Capsules containing concentrated eicosapentaenoic and docosahexaenoic oils have now appeared on the market and are variously recommended for the prevention of heart disease, hypertension, rheumatoid arthritis, and even migraine headaches. Although there is some experimental evidence to suggest that the Omega-3s can be of value in these conditions, you should not take these preparations before discussing it with your physician; they can have unwanted effects. For instance, although they may prevent blood clotting, by the same token they will increase the tendency to bleed excessively from minor cuts or scrapes, tooth extraction, or surgery. In susceptible individuals, or in those who are also taking aspirin as a blood thinner, this effect can be exaggerated. In diabetics, high doses of eicosapentaenoic oils can increase blood sugar levels and interfere with the action of insulin. Better by far, then, to get your Omega-3 oils the natural way — from fish.

Olive Oil

Ancel Keys found that monounsaturated fatty acid was neutral, whereas polyunsaturated fatty acid lowered cholesterol. This led to the recommendation that the latter be the preferred choice for the substitution of the saturated fatty acids in the diet. However, the commonest source of monounsaturated acid is olive oil, a major component of the Mediterranean diet for thousands of years. Since heart disease is less common in Mediterranean than Northern European countries, the feeling grew that olive oil must have something more to contribute than merely being neutral. This view seemed to be substantiated by a number of studies that suggested that, unlike the vegetable oils, which not only lower total cholesterol but may also reduce HDL-C, olive oil has no such undesirable effect on HDL-C. However, other reports have failed to confirm this. The jury is still out. On the basis that it has certainly stood the test of time, olive oil would not appear to have any harmful effects, but there is no strong scientific basis for preferring it over the vegetable oil linoleic acid as a substitute for saturated fatty acids. Its main benefit may be that it substitutes for animal fats in the Mediterranean diet.

DIET AND CHOLESTEROL

The Effects of Lowering Blood Cholesterol

The observation that a diet high in animal fat could cause hypercholesterolemia and eventually lead to coronary atherosclerosis has been put to the test by a series of prospective clinical trials. These fall into one of two categories, depending on whether the cholesterol lowering was attempted by altering the diet, or by giving a drug.

The three largest and most frequently quoted dietary trials were the Finnish Mental Hospital Study, the Los Angeles Veteran Study, and the Oslo Primary Prevention Trial. In total, they involved some 4,000 healthy men. All three showed that a diet low in animal fat resulted in a reduction in blood cholesterol levels, and this was associated with a significant drop in the incidence of fatal and non-fatal heart attacks. Despite these apparently impressive results, however, critics have pointed out that the conclusions would have been more convincing if more subjects had been included and if the design of the studies had been more scientific. They also note that apart from the Oslo Study, which included strategies to stop smoking, the overall death rates from all causes were the same in the diet and the control groups. In the case of the Veteran Study, the dieting group had an increase in deaths from cancer; this did not, however, reach statistically significant levels and thus could have been coincidental. Some additional support for critics of the low-fat diet comes from other reports, mostly in the British medical journals, of smaller but more scientifically controlled trials in which dietary intervention neither lowered cholesterol nor reduced heart attacks.

The use of drugs to test the cholesterol theory appears to have obvious advantages. It is easier to take a medication than to change one's diet, and therefore there is less of a problem with compliance. A placebo can be used for the control group, and the trial can be "blinded," that is, not only do the patients not know which group they are in, but neither do their doctors. This eliminates the possible influence of suggestion. The only drawback to be considered is the possibility of undesirable side effects from the drug.

This very problem of side effects did arise in connection with an early drug trial carried out by the World Health Organization in the 1960s and 1970s. The drug was successful in reducing cholesterol and non-fatal heart attacks. However, there were significantly more deaths in the treated group, due largely to increased incidence of gall bladder disease and intestinal cancer. While this could have been coincidental, one cannot ignore the possibility that it might have been a side effect of the drug.

The 1980s saw the results of two more drug trials, the American Lipid Research Clinic's Coronary Drug Prevention Trial, referred to simply as the LRC trial, and the Finnish Helsinki Trial. The former was the larger of the two, with approximately 4,000 hypercholesterolemic men divided into two groups, half receiving the cholesterol-lowering bile resin cholestyramine (Questran), and the other a placebo; the entire group was followed from 1973 to 1983. What was the outcome?

Now comes the difficult part. I could merely state that the majority of the medical profession, and particularly those who were involved in the trial, consider the results to be 100% conclusive evidence that hypercholesterolemia causes coronary atherosclerosis and that lowering high blood cholesterol levels prevents coronary atherosclerosis. There is strong *circumstantial* evidence to support that view, but on this matter I must admit to mixed feelings. I cannot in all conscience ignore the arguments of those scientists who take some exception to the majority interpretation of the LRC trial data. After all, I warned you at the outset of this book that I did not intend to sacrifice accuracy for simplicity. Ideally, the LRC trial should have shown a thoroughly convincing reduction in cholesterol levels and death from heart disease in the treated group. Physicians around the world were eagerly awaiting such an outcome. The facts that emerged were as follows: there were 38 deaths from heart attacks in the controls (2% of the group), and 30 (1.6%) in the treated group. This difference is not statistically significant. There were 158 non-fatal heart attacks in the controls (1.7%), and 130 (1.5%) in those treated. Again, this is not a statistically significant difference. On the other hand, if we add the fatal and the non-fatal attacks together, then we have 196 heart attacks in the controls (1.7%), and 160 in those treated (1.5%), and this difference is statistically significant, but only to the 0.05 level — i.e., there is a 5% chance of the difference being purely coincidental. The doubting Thomases insist that in a matter of such importance, the chances of coincidental findings should be no less than one in a hundred ($p = 0.01$), and preferably as little as one in a thousand ($p = 0.001$).

What do we make of all this? At first glance, the evidence in favor of cholesterol-lowering is not overwhelming, and certainly not as convincing or dramatic as one might have expected, given the earlier impressions from the Framingham and Seven Countries studies. Nevertheless, lowering cholesterol did have the desired effect in that it did reduce total heart attacks. Also, it should be recognized that the results of biological experiments are never as tidy and clear-cut as those encountered in the more exact sciences such as mathematics. As Dr. Lawrence Friedman, chief of the Clinical Trials Branch, National Heart, Lung, and Blood Institute, observed, "There is no such thing as a definitive clinical trial, the results of a clinical trial alone are not necessarily persuasive, nor should they be." By that, Dr. Friedman was underlining the fact that, while the LRC results were not thoroughly decisive, when added to all the knowledge gained from previous animal experiments and epidemiological studies, they powerfully reinforce the cholesterol argument. On balance, then, and despite detractors, my tendency is to accept that the LRC results do confirm the cholesterol theory.

Before leaving the LRC trial, we must mention one final nagging concern. Once again, as in the dietary studies, the total death rate was the same in the treated and untreated groups. The controls had 71 deaths (3%), and the treated 68 (3%). The reduction in heart attack fatalities was balanced by an increase in intestinal cancer and violent deaths.

The Helsinki trial involved 4,000 hypercholesterolemic males and the drug used was the triglyceride-lowering agent gemfibrozil (Lopid). This drug has the ability to increase HDL-cholesterol levels. As in the LRC study, there was no difference between the groups with regard to fatal or non-fatal heart attacks alone, but there was a significant difference when the two were added together. Death from all causes was the same in both groups, with slightly more violent deaths and incidence of cancer in the treated group.

Interpretation of Cholesterol-Lowering Trials
Out of all these trials and studies the following salient points emerge:

1. Reducing cholesterol levels in men with hypercholesterolemia reduces the incidence of combined fatal and non-fatal heart attacks.
2. This benefit is seen in the drug and the dietary intervention trials, although possibly not to the extent that might be expected from the Framingham and other predictions.

3. In addition to answering some questions, these trials have also posed others. Lowering cholesterol did not reduce the total number of deaths in the groups being studied. The reduction in coronary death was counterbalanced by an increase in death from intestinal disorders, cancer, and violent causes. These findings could be coincidental. However, violent deaths are consistently higher than the number occurring in the control groups and also higher than the national average.

4. Finally, dietary intervention has proven to be less consistent in lowering cholesterol level than drug therapy. If this finding is verified by future experience, does it mean that most of us will have to adopt a strict vegetarian diet (a move that would have severe economic and social consequences) or must we become candidates for lifelong cholesterol-lowering drugs? These concerns have prompted some members of the medical profession to question the application of the current cholesterol-lowering strategies to the population as a whole, and to recommend that they be reserved for high-risk individuals only.

Dealing with Hypercholesterolemia in the Population

Before we introduce any mass treatment strategy, we should be reasonably sure of its success and totally sure of its safety. Obviously, then, natural lifestyle changes such as eating prudently, exercising regularly, stopping smoking, and reducing obesity are preferable to drug therapy as preventive measures for the population as a whole. Drug therapy is better reserved for those who are at high risk, where the possible side effects outweigh the obvious benefits.

With these considerations in mind, we can proceed to the matter of detecting those who are at risk for heart disease because of elevated blood cholesterol and treating them accordingly. The first step in our strategy is to screen the population by making a blood test part of routine physical examinations. As a matter of fact, portable cholesterol analyzers now on the market give a reading from a finger-prick blood sample within two minutes, and in parts of the United States these are located in shopping centers, schools, and other public places in order to permit widespread screening.

Screening is only a means to an end. The next step is to identify a cholesterol level, or cut-off point, above which dietary guidance is indicated. More than 50% of fatal heart attacks occur in individuals who have cholesterol values between 200 mg/dL (5.2 mmol/L) and 240 mg/dL (6.2 mmol/L) *and also possess two or more of the other major risk factors*, or who have evidence of coronary disease, i.e., a previous heart attack or angina. On the other hand, people *without any risk factors* and with cholesterol values below 240 mg/dL (6.2 mmol/L) have only a minimal risk of heart disease. With this in mind, we can better appreciate the thinking behind the cholesterol-lowering guidelines outlined by the American National Cholesterol Education Program (NCEP) that have been adopted, with minor modifications, in practically all countries where coronary disease is a problem. Cholesterol levels below 200 mg/dL (5.2 mmol/L) are considered to be "desirable." Levels above 200 mg/dL (5.2 mmol/L) but below 240 mg/dL (6.2 mmol/L) are classified as "borderline," and those above this as "high." Obviously, those individuals who fall into the desirable category will require no further action, apart from a repeat cholesterol reading in, say, five years' time. Those at high risk will be entered into a dietary and/or drug program. However, 25% of the adult population will be borderline (5.2 mmol/L to 6.2 mmol/L), and in North America alone this group will comprise many millions. Before being considered for intervention, these people should undergo a second screening consisting of a more complete blood test at a medical laboratory to determine LDL-C and HDL-C levels, and a check for a history of coronary disease, or the presence of other major risk factors (male sex, a family history of coronary heart disease at an early age, cigarette smoking, high blood pressure, diabetes, and obesity). The NCEP recommends dietary modification as the first step in intervention; drug therapy should be considered only after six months of careful dieting, and even then only if the LDL-C remains above the recommended level. The guidelines are shown in Appendix H.

Multiple Risk Factors

The NCEP strategy, while concentrating on cholesterol levels, illustrates the powerful cumulative effect of additional risk factors (Figure 22). What may be less obvious is the multiplicative effect of the presence of a number of risk factors that are only mildly elevated. For instance, an individual with a mildly elevated blood cholesterol of 240 mg/dL (6.2 mmol/L), and a borderline-high diastolic blood pressure of 100 mm Hg, who smokes only five cigarettes a day, might be considered to be at low risk; in fact, the risk would be as high as that for someone with a blood cholesterol of 300 mg/dL (7.8 mmol/L) or a diastolic blood pressure of 110 mm Hg, or who smokes two packs of cigarettes a day! (Figure 23.)

Multiple Risk Factor Intervention

A series of clinical trials has attempted to put this knowledge to good use. So far, we have dealt with each risk factor separately, whether it be hypercholesterolemia, hypertension, or cigarette smoking. However, from what we have learned, it seems naive to believe that we can reduce the incidence of a multi-factorial disease by attacking one risk factor only. We are clearly more likely to achieve success by using a broader multi-factorial approach. How have we fared in this regard?

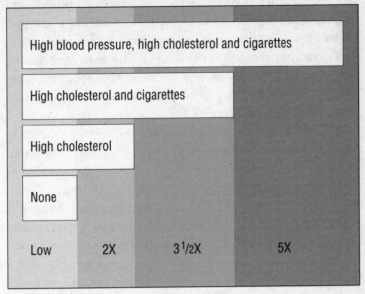

Figure 22: *Cumulative Effect of Additional Risk Factors*
The individual who exhibits multiple risk factors greatly increases the chance of developing coronary disease.

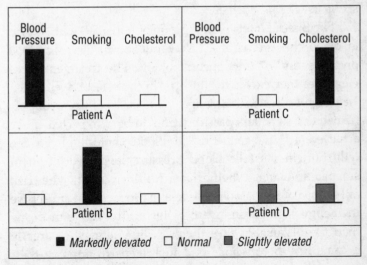

Figure 23: *Balancing Risk Factors*
Four patients, A, B, C and D have the same risk of developing coronary disease. In the case of patients A, B and C, the presence of one markedly elevated risk factor is obvious. Patient D, with three mildly elevated factors, may not recognize the extent of the risk.

The Multiple Risk Factor Intervention Study was launched by the American National Heart and Lung Institute in the 1970s, and its results were first published in 1982. It is usually referred to as the MRFIT. This is an unfortunate acronym, since it had nothing to do with fitness or exercise, except, as you will see in the next chapter, as an after-thought. The MRFIT involved 22 medical centers around the United States, cost about $15 million, and is an excellent example of how the best-laid plans can go wrong. The study design called for the enrollment of some 12,000 middle-aged healthy men who were at risk for coronary disease because of hypercholesterolemia, hypertension, and ciga-rette smoking. The treatment control group, to be known as the Special Intervention group, received intensive smok-ing and dietary counselling as well as treatment of the hypertension. The control or Usual Care group was given an annual physical check-up, but otherwise was left to its own devices. All subjects were informed of their risk factors at the commencement of the trial, which was to last for six years.

The Special Intervention group obtained a 7% reduction in blood cholesterol, an 11.5% reduction in diastolic blood pressure, and 67% stopped smoking. The treatment goals were thus met, except for the drop in cholesterol level, which was slightly less than anticipated. The Usual Care subjects turned out to be less passive than had been expected. They achieved a 5.2% reduction in blood cholesterol, an 8% reduction in diastolic blood pressure, and 54% of them stopped smoking. Whether as a result of joining the trial, or because of increased public health propaganda, or because their family physicians were better at preventive medicine than the organizers gave them credit for, they apparently became health conscious and took steps to improve their coronary profile. Thus, at the end of the six years, the coronary death rates were almost identical.

Since MRFIT did not achieve what it intended — that is, to show a significantly lower coronary mortality in the Special Intervention group — it is considered by some to be a failed trial. The fact that there were so few deaths in both groups suggests that the selection criteria may have been too stringent, resulting in the inadvertent selection of men with a lower than expected coronary mortality. The simplest explanation, of course, is that the substantial reduction in at least two of the three risk factors by the Usual Care group contributed to its low death rate, thus indicating the advantage of multiple risk reduction.

The residents of the county of North Karelia in East Finland had one of the highest death rates from coronary artery disease in the world. In the 1960s, they asked their government to do something about it. As a result, the North Karelia Project was instituted. A baseline screening assessment showed that more than half the subjects in the study were smokers and suffered from hypercholesterolemia and hypertension. As a result, an intensive community program was implemented, integrating all the health and social services of the country. Over the period 1969 to 1979, North Karelia reported a 24% decline in coronary mortality in men and a 51% decline in women. The investigators concluded that this impressive reduction in coronary disease was convincing proof of the value of community risk factor reduction.

These trials indicate the potential benefits of the multi-risk factor reduction approach. They also demonstrate that strategies involving lifestyle interventions do not produce harmful side effects.

What about Exercise?
The studies and trials I have referred to so far do not appear to have addressed the matter of physical activity and its relationship to heart disease. Actually, the Seven Countries

Study used a single multiple-choice question to divide individuals into sedentary, moderately active, and very active. When one considers the limited nature of such an enquiry, the diverse pattern of cultures under study, and the difficulty in defining physical activity levels in such widely different societies, it is not surprising that the results were inconclusive. Similarly, the Framingham Study gathered only limited information on physical activity patterns, although it was sufficient for the principal investigators to come to the conclusion that regular exercise, even at a minimal intensity, did contribute to a reduced CHD incidence. Dr. William Kannel, the pioneering physician whose vision gave rise to the Framingham Study, later agreed that a more searching evaluation of physical activity habits might have been even more productive. His colleague, Dr. William Castelli, also a firm advocate of the cholesterol theory, is fair-minded (or pragmatic) enough to include jogging as part of his weekly routine. We will look at the benefits of physical activity later, but in the meantime let us see how we diagnose and treat coronary heart disease.

5. Detection and Treatment

The classic symptoms and signs of angina pectoris and of a heart attack are well known. Any patient who arrives at a doctor's office or an emergency department of a hospital with these symptoms is usually swiftly diagnosed. However, various tests are needed to confirm the diagnosis, particularly when the symptoms are not typical.

The Electrocardiogram

The ECG (or, in America, the EKG) is the most frequently used cardiac diagnostic test. It consists of a tracing of the minute amounts of electrical activity generated by the heart muscle when it contracts. Electrodes, small metal plates, are placed on the body to record the electrical current from different parts of the heart. Usually there are ten electrodes, one over each wrist and above each ankle, and six placed across the front of the chest. These give us an electrical picture of the beating heart as viewed from its front, back, and bottom surface. For convenience, each deflection, or wave, of the tracing is labelled by the consecutive letters P, Q, R, S, and T (Figure 24). The first deflection, the P wave, is caused by the upper chambers of the heart, the atria, contracting. Thereafter, there is a short pause while

Figure 24: Normal Electrocardiogram Showing ST Segment

the current passes to the lower chambers, the ventricles. When the ventricles contract, they give rise to the QRS wave or complex. After another delay, there is a further flow of current, which re-charges the heart and prepares it for its next beat; the re-charge results in the T wave. The interval between the end of the QRS complex and the beginning of the T wave is referred to as the ST segment and is very important in modern cardiology. If the shape, particularly the angle, of its slope changes during exercise when the heart is beating rapidly, it can be a very early sign of coronary disease.

A heart attack gives rise to characteristic abnormalities in the ECG tracing. These changes may take some hours to develop after the onset of symptoms, but usually they are easily recognizable, even in their early stages. The part of the heart that has been damaged by the attack can be identified by the electrode or group of electrodes showing the greatest abnormalities. Heart attack ECG changes are generally permanent, since the scar tissue, although it functions satisfactorily, never regains the normal pattern of electrical activity. Anginal pain, since it does not cause permanent damage to heart muscle cells, can be detected on the ECG only at the time of the attack, and even then not consistently. The commonest type of irregularity met with is extrasystoles, or "skipped beats" (see Chapter 10).

The Exercise Test
We have seen that a person can suffer from coronary artery disease for many years before developing angina. Since anginal symptoms are frequently brought on by exercise, recognition of the disease is delayed even further if the person never exercises. By the time the usual low-level activities of daily living give rise to symptoms, the degree of coronary atherosclerosis is usually quite severe. However, if we can have the subject exercise at gradually increasing intensities of effort, we may be able to induce typical anginal pain even when the degree of coronary narrowing is quite moderate and the presence of disease otherwise unrecognized. The exercise test is usually performed on a treadmill or a stationary cycle. The subject is connected to an electrocardiogram, so that a continuous ECG tracing is obtained throughout the test. The speed of the treadmill belt at the start of the test is quite slow, about 2 miles (3 kilometers) per hour. The angulation, or slope, is set at zero. Every two or three minutes, the speed and slope are increased slightly. The initial stages call for a slow easy stroll, gradually progressing to vigorous uphill jogging. If the cycle is used, the level of effort is increased by adjusting the pedal resistance every minute. The test is supervised or actually carried out by a physician, assisted by nursing and exercise laboratory staff. The person exercises until forced to stop because of extreme leg fatigue and breathlessness. The length of time of the test may vary from

nine to fifteen minutes, depending on the subject's fitness level. In the case of a coronary patient, the test is often stopped by the physician because of the onset of angina. In this case, a test is referred to as being a "symptom limited maximal test."

However, the exercise test's major contribution to the early diagnosis of coronary disease comes not just from the detection of anginal pain, but from the fact that it allows us to see changes that occur in the simultaneously recorded exercise ECG *before* the onset of angina. Indeed, these changes may even take place in the *absence* of anginal pain, in which case they are referred to as "silent angina" or, more recently in medical parlance, "silent ischaemia." The abnormalities referred to involve the ST segment. This part of the tracing becomes increasingly depressed as the blood flow through the coronary arteries becomes more restricted (Figure 25). When a coronary-prone patient develops exercise chest pain of uncertain origin accompanied by ST segment depression, we can be almost completely certain that this pain is due to coronary disease. The earlier in the test, and therefore the lower the level of effort at which the pain and/or the ST segment changes occur, the more severe the degree of coronary narrowing. Of course, no medical test is 100% accurate. There are rare occasions when ST depression is due to some other cause (for example, the drug digitalis, or abnormal electrical pathways in the heart, situations with which the physician will be thoroughly familiar). Nevertheless, a positive exercise test in a patient with a strong family history of coronary disease or one who possesses two or more coronary risk factors usually indicates the presence of atherosclerosis.

In addition to ST segment changes, the exercise ECG can also detect the presence of effort-induced irregular heartbeats, which, if they become too frequent, can be another indication to halt the test. Blood pressure is also monitored every two minutes so as to see that it is

Figure 25: Electrocardiogram Indicating Coronary Disease
(A) Normal electrocardiogram at rest, and (B) showing depression of ST segment during exercise indicating restriction of blood flow through the coronary arteries.

responding normally to exercise. Finally, we can collect and analyze the subject's expired breath throughout the test. This enables us to measure the amount of oxygen being used at peak effort, giving us the maximum oxygen intake, or VO_2max, an excellent measure of cardiovascular fitness. From this we can calculate a safe and effective exercise training intensity. Furthermore, using the information obtained from this analysis, we can construct a graph showing how the breathing rate increases with each stage of the test. We will then be able to see a point at which the subject's breathing starts to become more rapid and labored. This point signifies the early onset of fatigue and lactic acid build-up and is referred to as the anaerobic threshold (Figure 26). It corresponds to about 60% of the peak oxygen intake, and a level of 12 to 14 on the Borg Scale of Perceived Exertion (Figure 34), and is a further cor-roboration of the correct training intensity. Collection of ex-

Figure 26: Anaerobic Threshold
The anaerobic threshold is the point at which the relationship between breathing and exercise becomes non-linear. This is an appropriate level of exertion for endurance training.

pired air is carried out through a mouthpiece connected by flexible hosing to a sophisticated machine that analyzes the breath for oxygen and carbon dioxide content. Leakage of air through the nose is prevented by the use of a nose clip. Since cardiac departments are interested more in detecting coronary disease than in prescribing exercise, they usually dispense with this equipment. However, it is used at the Toronto Rehabilitation Centre.

OTHER METHODS OF INVESTIGATING THE HEART

Echocardiography
High-frequency sound waves are generated by an ultrasonic machine and are "bounced" off the heart; these sound echoes are then converted into electrical energy to display a moving

image on an oscilloscope screen. Thus, one can determine the size of the heart's chambers, the thickness of its walls, and the efficiency of its performance. If the examination is done before and immediately after exercise, one is even better able to detect abnormalities in the heart's pumping capacity. There is no radioactivity involved, and the patient feels nothing during the examination.

Radionuclide Imaging

This procedure involves the use of radioactive substances called radio isotopes, which are injected into the bloodstream through a vein in the arm and then detected in the body by a highly sensitive Gamma camera. Two types of tests are in common use. In the first, radionuclide ventriculography, an isotope called technetium is attached to the red cells, and pictures are taken of the blood pool within the chambers of the heart, particularly the ventricles. The amount of blood ejected with each beat can be seen and the pumping efficiency assessed accordingly. In the second, the isotope called thallium is used. It is carried through the coronary arteries to the walls of the heart. If blood flow is reduced in a particular coronary artery branch because of atherosclerotic narrowing, the camera will show little or no thallium in the portion of the wall supplied by the narrowed artery. This type of imaging is usually combined with an exercise test, which emphasizes its effect and can be helpful in doubtful cases of effort-induced angina or ST segment depression. The radio isotopes used in these tests have very short half-lives, which means they are cleared very rapidly from the body. They are also used in such minute quantities that they do not constitute any danger to the patient.

Telemetry

This test consists of radio transmission of the ECG to a receiver-printer. It permits an ECG in situations where solid wire connecting cables between the patient and the ECG machine would be impractical, for example, when the patient is walking or jogging. In the cardiac rehabilitation setting, it is used to monitor patients for the presence of exercise-induced ST segment depression or skipped beats, usually during workouts or simulated job tasks. It is also used to check the patient's ability to take a pulse accurately. The transmission range is usually up to 110 yards (100 meters), provided there are no obstructions between the patient and the receiver.

Ambulatory Electrocardiogram Monitoring

This technique is used to detect ECG abnormalities that are suspected to be occurring during activities of daily living and while away from the hospital or doctor's office. Chest electrodes are connected to a small tape recorder that is strapped to the waist. The apparatus is usually worn for 24 hours, during which time the patient keeps an activity diary, recording any unusual symptoms. When the tape is returned, it is run through a computerized rapid analyzer, which detects any irregularities and relates them to the comments on the diary.

Cardiac Catheterization (Coronary Angiography)

Unlike the previous tests, this one is "invasive." A thin hollow tube, or catheter, is carefully pushed through a small cut in a thigh or arm artery and then threaded up the vessel and on into the aorta until its tip lies opposite the openings of the coronary arteries. The procedure is carried out by a cardiologist, who carefully watches the passage of the catheter on an X-ray display. Once the tip of the catheter is in position, a dye that is visible on the X-ray is injected into all three coronary arteries and its flow observed on a large video screen; the pictures are also recorded on film for subsequent playback and re-examination (Figure 27). As the dye passes down the coronary vessels, one can see

Figure 27: Angiogram
An angiogram X-ray of coronary arteries showing narrowing (see arrow) in the upper portion of the anterior descending branch of the left coronary artery.

any narrowing or obstruction. The procedure causes only minor discomfort (a hot "flush" as the dye is being injected), but the patient has to keep the affected leg or arm still for about six hours after the procedure so as to prevent bleeding from the incision. Nowadays there is an increasing tendency for cardiac catheterization to be carried out on an out-patient basis.

The risks of catheterization are minimal, but the most serious includes precipitating a fatal heart attack. While the chances of this are only about one in a thousand or even less, catheterization is not carried out except in situations where angioplasty or coronary artery bypass surgery are being seriously considered. Certainly mere curiosity as to the degree of coronary disease is not a usual indication.

MEDICATIONS FREQUENTLY USED IN THE TREATMENT OF CORONARY DISEASE

There are a number of drugs used in the treatment of coronary heart disease. The commonest groups are appropriately discussed here.

Nitrates

This group of drugs is used to treat angina. They act by opening up, or dilating, the veins and arteries (including the coronaries) throughout the body, thus reducing the work load on the heart and improving its blood supply. They come in a number of preparations. The short-acting nitroglycerine tablet is placed under the tongue until it dissolves; its effect is lost if it is swallowed. It relieves anginal pain quickly, usually within a minute or so, and the relief lasts for up to an hour. It can cause a throbbing headache, or even fainting in some people. These side effects lessen with use. It can also prevent angina if taken before exercise.

Nitroglycerine tablets deteriorate with time and should be replaced after about two months. Their strength declines more rapidly if they are stored in a plastic container with cotton batting, or carried in a pants' pocket. Better to keep them in a glass bottle with a foil-lined cap.

Nitroglycerine aerosol sprays are now in common use, the usual dose being one or two puffs. Adhesive skin patches are yet another form of delivering the drug. They are usually applied over the chest and are intended to maintain a constant level of nitroglycerine in the blood. However, it has been established that tolerance, with loss of anti-anginal effect, can develop with continuous nitrate administration. Apparently this is prevented by intermittent use. Therefore, if patches are used, they are generally removed for a time during a 24-hour period, usually during the night. Long-acting nitrate is given in the form of isosorbide dinitrate (trade name Isordil); unlike the nitroglycerine tablet, it is not destroyed by the internal digestive juices, so it can be swallowed. The anti-anginal effect lasts four to six hours and may be prescribed three or four times a day.

Beta-adrenoreceptor-blocker (beta-blockers)

The increase in heart rate and blood pressure that accompanies the body's "fight or flight" response is brought about by the action of the hormones adrenaline and noradrenaline on small, button-like structures, called beta-adrenoreceptors, that are located throughout the heart muscle. Beta-blockers prevent or block the entry of these hormones into the receptors and so cancel out their stimulating effect. Thus, they reduce the speed and force of the heartbeat, that is, the pulse rate and blood pressure. Beta-blockers are used in the treatment of the following conditions: (i) exercise- or stress-induced angina, because they reduce the work of the heart; (ii) hypertension, because they reduce blood pressure; (iii) certain types of irregular heartbeats (skipped beats); (iv) heart attack, in selected cases, in order to prevent a recurrence; (v) glaucoma, in the form of eye drops, because they lower the pressure inside the eye; (vi) migraine, because they prevent the blood vessels in the brain from over-dilating; and (vii) occasionally to calm nerves or tremor in public speakers or actors on "first nights," or professional sportsmen such as marksmen, musicians, or pool players.

There are a few real contraindications to the use of beta-blockers. They may not be suitable for patients suffering from severe asthma, bronchitis, or other forms of lung disease, because they block the beta receptors in the lungs that, as part of the noradrenaline effect, open up the airways so as to receive more oxygen. They are also not good for patients who suffer from peripheral vascular disease, in which atherosclerosis has reduced the circulation of blood to the legs, because they can cause cold feet and hands. Beta-blockers are not advisable for patients who are suffering from heart failure, since by reducing pumping power they aggravate the condition. They can also interfere with glucose metabolism and are used only with great caution in insulin-dependent diabetics.

Although small doses of a beta-blocker may not affect heart rate, larger doses invariably will, and allowance must be made for this when using pulse rates as a guide in exercise training. This will be dealt with more fully in Chapter 10.

Some beta-blockers in large doses may hinder full utilization by the skeletal muscle of its major fuels, fat and starch, and in this way cause early muscle fatigue. The exerciser may suddenly become tired during a workout and have to stop because of leg fatigue. Where this problem is excessive, improvement may be obtained by switching to another beta-blocker, one that has less peripheral effect. Other side effects may include diarrhea, nausea, depression, loss of sexual urge, and reduction of HDL-cholesterol.

Finally, beta-blockers should not be stopped suddenly after they have been used for a prolonged period of time. This can result in a sudden over-sensitivity to noradrenaline, with consequent swift return of symptoms such as severe angina or marked elevation of blood pressure. There have even been reports of heart attacks occurring after sudden cessation of a beta-blocker. Where the medication has to be stopped, it should be done gradually and under the supervision of your physician.

Since they were first introduced in 1956, many new beta-blockers have been developed. They differ from each other only insofar as they might act primarily to relieve angina, or lower blood pressure, or both, or in whether they are long or short acting, or in the manner in which they bring about various minor side effects in different individuals. The choice can be made only by the physician. The most commonly prescribed go under the trade names of Inderal (propranolol), Blocadren (timolol), Corgard (nadolol), Sotacor (sotalol), Sectral (acebutolol), Tenormin (atenolol),

Lopressor (metoprolol), Visken (pindolol), and Trandate (labetalol).

Calcium Channel Blockers

This class of heart drug was introduced in 1976 and was approved for use in heart disease in North America in the 1980s. It acts by slowing the rate at which calcium moves backwards and forwards across the walls of the cells via special passages called calcium channels. Slowing the passage of calcium reduces the force with which the cells work. The effect on heart muscle cells is to lessen the force and speed of the heart's contractions, thus reducing cardiac work load. The arteries of the body, including the coronary arteries, respond to the calcium channel blockers by relaxing. Calcium channel blockers are therefore used to treat angina and also hypertension. Because they relax the muscular walls of the coronary arteries, they are unique in their ability to treat a particular type of angina known as Prinzmetal's angina, which occurs at rest, and is due to a spasm of the coronary arteries. The cause of the condition is unknown; it may even occur in those whose coronary arteries are free from atherosclerosis, and, as I have said, until the introduction of the calcium channel blockers, it was a major treatment problem. The most common calcium channel blockers used in North America go under the trade names of Isoptin (verapamil), Cardene (nicardipine), Cardizem (diltiazem), and Adalat (nifedipine). Each has a slightly different action, and, as in the beta-blockers, your physician will choose whichever is most suitable in your case.

Digitalis

Derived originally from the leaf of the common purple foxglove, digitalis, or digoxin, has been used by physicians for many years. Since its main purpose is to strengthen the heart's action, it is used in heart failure. Digitalis accumulates in the body, and it may take as long as two weeks after its use is discontinued for its effect on the heart rate to disappear — an important fact if the physician stops the drug temporarily for the purpose of checking progress by means of an exercise test. Digitalis can cause a false depression of the ST segment of the electrocardiogram, both at rest and during an exercise test. It also tends to slow the resting heart rate.

DRUGS THAT REDUCE TENDENCY OF BLOOD TO CLOT PLATELET INHIBITORS

Aspirin

In its natural form, salicylic acid, aspirin is obtained from the bark of various species of the willow and poplar. Today it is used in its synthesized form, acetylsalicylic acid. The humble aspirin has been used by physicians since the days of ancient Greece. It is still used extensively to reduce fever, relieve pain, reduce inflammation, and treat arthritis. It leapt into prominence in the context of coronary heart disease when it was discovered that it was a mild anti-clotting agent. It acts by inhibiting the first steps in the formation of a blood clot, which is the clumping together of the blood platelet cells and then the sticking of these clumps to the inner wall of an artery. Since this process is often the first stage in the development of a heart attack, this discovery led to a series of clinical trials to determine if aspirin could (i) reduce the death rate from a heart attack in its early stages shortly after the onset, (ii) reduce the likelihood of a recurrent heart attack, (iii) reduce the likelihood of a future heart attack in patients suffering from severe unstable angina, and (iv) prevent a first heart attack in healthy individuals who are apparently free from coronary disease.

The answer given by the various studies to the first three questions is an unqualified yes.

Obviously, in these situations, aspirin is given by prescription and at the discretion of the patient's physician. The latter will take into account the fact that aspirin does, however, have some undesirable side effects. It is a well-known gastric irritant and can lead to peptic ulcers or cause them to bleed. People with a strong family or personal history of hemorrhagic stroke (a type caused by a blood vessel bursting and bleeding into the brain tissue) probably should not take aspirin at all.

What about the use of aspirin in healthy individuals in order to protect them from heart disease? Here the evidence is more conflicting. In essence, we have two studies, one American and one British, which appear to contradict one another. The American study involved 22,000 male physicians. Half were assigned to take one 325-mg aspirin tablet every other day, while the other half were given an aspirin-free placebo. At the end of five years, it was found that the aspirin takers had about 45% fewer heart attacks than the non-aspirin takers. The news was so good that it was released to the media and proclaimed around the world before other physicians and medical scientists had a chance to review the data in detail. However, a British study, also using male physicians, although smaller in size and using a slightly higher dose of aspirin (500 mg daily) found no advantage in terms of fatal or non-fatal heart attacks to the aspirin takers. Both studies, however, did show that taking aspirin was associated with a higher incidence of hemorrhagic stroke and bleeding ulcers. Admittedly, the numbers who suffered these side effects were not large enough to be statistically significant, but they are nevertheless disturbing.

There is one aspect of the American study that is of interest. The American physicians, unlike the British, seemed a remarkably healthy lot. A large group of males of that age group (40-84 years) would have been expected to experience a considerable number of deaths from heart

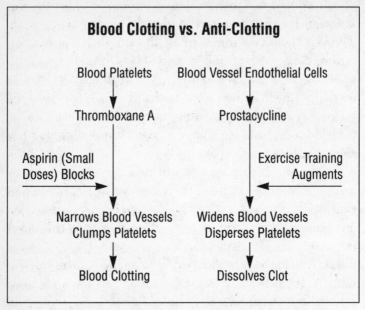

Blood Clotting vs. Anti-Clotting

Blood Platelets   Blood Vessel Endothelial Cells

Thromboxane A   Prostacycline

Aspirin (Small
Doses) Blocks   Exercise Training
                       Augments

Narrows Blood Vessels   Widens Blood Vessels
Clumps Platelets   Disperses Platelets

Blood Clotting   Dissolves Clot

Figure 28: The Interaction Between Blood Platelets and Blood Vessel Endothelial Cells in Blood Clot Formation

disease over the five-year period. In fact, there were only 36 fatal and 342 non-fatal heart attacks in the group of 22,000 subjects. In addition, of the total group, 72% exercised vigorously at least once a week, only 11% smoked, and 82% had total cholesterol levels of less than 5.2 mmol/L!

What can we make of all this? Firstly, there is the question of dosage. The American trial used a 325-mg tablet every other day, whereas the British study used 500 mg every day. It could be that the higher doses of aspirin not only block the action of Thromboxane A, which causes platelets to clump together, but also the formation of Prostacycline, the substance produced by the endothelium, which prevents the platelets from sticking to one another and to the blood vessel wall (Figure 28).

Also, the greatest decrease in heart attacks occurred in the American physicians aged 50 years and older; there was no difference in the number of heart attacks in those under the age of 50, whether or not they took aspirin. As for sudden cardiac death, a common occurrence in those suffering from coronary heart disease, aspirin did not reduce this. With regard to total cardiovascular deaths (heart attacks, sudden cardiac death, and strokes added together), this was almost identical in the two groups — 81 deaths in the aspirin takers and 83 in the controls.

If you do not suffer from coronary heart disease, but are thinking of taking aspirin as a preventative, I advise you to discuss this with your doctor first. If you are over 50, have a family history of coronary heart disease, and the other risk factors are being attended to, then a reasonable approach might be to take a small dose of aspirin, even as low as 80 mg every day or every second day. The lower the dose, the less the likelihood of side effects. At the same time, it appears that even low doses can have a good anti-platelet effect. If there is a history of hemorrhagic stroke in the family, then you should tell your physician. Also, remember that bleeding is prolonged by aspirin usage, and this can be a problem during surgery, even minor surgery, or dental procedures. In the meantime, research is continuing, and it should not be too long before we can adopt a more definitive approach.

ANTICOAGULANTS

This group of drugs has no effect on platelets, but prevents clotting by interfering with the formation of fibrin, the protein strands that bind the clot together. They are potent anti-clotting substances and are prescribed only under strict medical supervision, which includes regular laboratory tests to see that the blood is not becoming too thin.

Warfarin (Coumadin) is the most frequently used oral anticoagulant. It is given for a three- to six-month period after the heart attack in those cases where troublesome clotting has occurred during the hospital stay, or where, because of the nature of the damage to the heart, clotting might be expected to occur within the walls or chambers after hospital discharge. Because of the great caution and care that must be exercised to maintain a safe and effective dosage, routine long-term use of warfarin to prevent another heart attack is now rarely practiced. Aspirin is safer and probably just as effective. However, warfarin is frequently used after open heart surgery where an artificial valve is inserted, to prevent clot formation on its surface.

Fibrinolytics (thrombolytics) are the so-called wonder drugs of the 1980s. Because they dissolve the fibrin strands in the blood clot, they are also referred to as "clot busters." Administered by intravenous injection within the first few hours after the onset of a heart attack, they break up the clot in the coronary artery, restore normal blood flow, and prevent damage to heart muscle. A number of large-scale international clinical trials have demonstrated that their use reduces the risk of death from heart attack by as much as 50%. The two drugs currently in use are streptokinase and tissue plasminogen activator (t-PA).

t-PA is of considerable interest, since it is a natural clot-buster produced by the body, and I will refer later to the fact that exercise training enhances its production. Initially, for large-scale treatment purposes it was of academic interest only, since, because it had to be extracted from human tissue, it was only available in very small quantities. It can now be manufactured by the process of genetic engineering to give recombinant tissue plasminogen activator (rt-PA).

A current problem with fibrinolytic therapy is the reformation of clot after discontinuing the drug. This occurs in about 5% to 20% of cases, but evidence suggests that this figure may be reduced if an injectable anticoagulant drug, heparin, is given concurrently. At the moment, trials are continuing to test new substances, or the effect of combination therapy, e.g., streptokinase plus rt-PA, with or without aspirin. The future of these agents is very exciting and promising.

CHOLESTEROL-LOWERING DRUGS

These fall into four broad categories: the bile resins, the fibrates, the cholesterol inhibitors, and niacin.

The Bile Resins
The commonest in use are cholestyramine (Questran) and colestipol (Colestid). These come in the form of granules, either in bulk, or more conveniently, in one-dose packages. They are mixed with water and taken with meals. The resins are not absorbed into the bloodstream but pass unaltered through the gut. Their action is to increase the excretion of bile and cholesterol in the stools. The side effects include gas, bloating, and constipation, but these tend to lessen with continued use.

The Fibrates
The commonest are clofibrate (Atromid-S) and gemfibrozil (Lopid); both come in capsule form and are taken by mouth. These have some cholesterol-lowering effect, but are more effective in reducing triglycerides. In a number of large-scale clinical trials, clofibrate has been found to increase the incidence of gall bladder disease and gallstones and for this reason is now less frequently used.

The Cholesterol Inhibitors
This new group of drugs prevents the liver from making cholesterol. The commonest in use are lovastatin (Mevacor), simvastatin (Zocor), and pravastatin (Pravachol). These are the most powerful cholesterol-lowering drugs available. They are taken with the evening meal, or before going to bed, since cholesterol manufacture takes place mainly

during sleeping hours. Preliminary studies show that these drugs have relatively few side effects, although long-term trials are still lacking. Rarely they can cause damage to the liver and the peripheral muscles, and for this reason the manufacturers advise regular blood tests to-check for this, particularly in the early months of treatment. New and improved members of the group will undoubtedly appear in the near future. These substances well may become the future drugs of choice in cases of hypercholesterolemia that are resistant to other measures.

Niacin

Otherwise known as Vitamin B3, nicotinic acid, or nicotinamide, niacin is found naturally in liver, lean meat, poultry, fish, whole grains, beans, and nuts. In the 1950s, it was found that if it was given in large doses, 1 to 2 grams or more daily, it could lower LDL-cholesterol and also raise HDL-cholesterol.

There is an obvious appeal to using a naturally occurring substance such as a vitamin to cure or prevent heart disease. Unfortunately, the benefit is more apparent than real. Vitamins given in mega doses are drugs and as such can have unpleasant side effects. The fact that they can be bought over the counter in any drugstore or health food store may make them even more of a potential hazard. In doses in excess of 250 milligrams, the side effects of niacin are more irritating than dangerous and include flushing of the skin, tingling, itching, and headache. In most cases, these can be avoided by building up to the larger doses gradually, taking niacin with food, or taking an aspirin an hour or so before the niacin tablet. However, doses of niacin in the order of 1 to 2 grams or more daily can have more serious side effects. Gastric irritation is not uncommon, and peptic ulcers may be aggravated. Blood sugar levels can be increased, which can pose a major problem for the very individuals who often suffer from hypercholesterolemia, i.e., Type II diabetics. A more serious problem involves the use of the sustained-release or long-acting niacin, which was developed in order to prevent the flushing and tingling that occurred with the short-acting tablet. Unfortunately, it seems that the long-acting form can be more toxic to the liver, and a number of cases have been reported of individuals who have developed liver damage after taking 2 to 4 grams of sustained-release niacin daily over a period of months.

You should take niacin to reduce blood cholesterol only under the direction of a physician. In that way, not only will your cholesterol be monitored every six months or so, but you can also have blood glucose and liver function tests carried out at the same time.

It should be stressed that all these drugs have side effects and should be used only after a trial of low-fat diet, weight reduction, and exercise has failed to reduce elevated cholesterol levels.

DRUGS USED FOR HEART FAILURE AND/OR HYPERTENSION

Diuretics, commonly referred to as "water pills," help the body to lose excess water and salt by increasing urine flow. This action prevents "waterlogging" of the legs and ankles, as well as the lungs, which occurs as a result of heart failure. The loss of water from the blood also reduces the total blood volume, which in turn causes the pressure to drop in the blood vessels. Thus diuretics are also used to treat hypertension. Diuretics can have some undesirable side effects, all of which can, fortunately, easily be prevented. One of the most serious is the loss of too much potassium from the body; it passes out in the urine together with the sodium in the salt. Not enough potassium causes weakness and can also trigger irregular heart rhythm in the form of skipped beats. To avoid these, potassium supplements can be taken in the form of potassium pills or fresh fruit and vegetables, which are rich in potassium. Alternatively your doctor can prescribe a special type of potassium-sparing diuretic that does not cause potassium loss. Other side effects include a disturbance in the way the body metabolizes glucose, and therefore diabetes may be a contraindication. Some diuretics given over a prolonged period of time can cause attacks of gout. Finally, they may also increase blood triglycerides and reduce HDL-cholesterol levels; these undesirable changes can, however, be offset by diet and exercise.

There are numerous diuretics on the market, but the most commonly used are hydrochlorothiazide (HydroDiuril, Aldactazide), furosemide (Lasix), chlorthalidone (Hygroton), and triamterene (Dyazide); the last is an example of a "potassium sparer."

Angiotensin-Converting Enzyme (ACE) Inhibitors
This group of drugs prevents the formation in the body of a substance called angiotensin, the action of which is to constrict the arteries. ACE inhibitors allow the blood vessels to dilate, thereby dropping the blood pressure and relieving the load on a heart. These agents are playing an increasingly successful role in treatment of heart disease, and many more are in the process of development. The three most common in use now are captopril (Capoten), enalapril (Vasotec), and lisinopril (Prinivil). Side effects are seldom serious, but the most troublesome is a dry irritating cough, which can lead to discontinuing the drug; others include an excessive drop in blood pressure, kidney problems, and elevated blood potassium levels.

6. Can Physical Activity Prevent Heart Disease?

If time travel were possible, a visitor from a bygone age to the twentieth century would surely be impressed by the extent to which we have eliminated physical activity from our daily routine. Modern transportation methods have made walking almost entirely a leisure activity. The elevator and the escalator save us from climbing steps. Automation is the order of the day in the factory and on the farm. Television keeps us tied to our favorite chair during the evenings and weekends. As if that isn't enough, we now have golf courses that display the sign "No walking permitted: golfers must use electric carts provided"! The United States Department of Health has estimated that whereas at the turn of the century more than 30% of all the energy expended by the workforce came from muscular effort, this figure had dropped to less than 1% by the mid-twentieth century.

Human beings have been civilized only within the last 10,000 years; for 1 million years before we discovered that we could grow and eat grain (provided we stayed around long enough to reap it), we were nomads and hunters. We moved with the game, walking, running, stalking, and constantly setting up and breaking camp. Is 10,000 years long enough to extinguish the needs of our bodies for activity and motion? If it were, why is the child still afraid of the dark? Why does our hair stand on end and why do our pupils dilate in preparation for fight or flight when we are startled? We are closer to our Stone Age ancestors than we sometimes choose to admit. If we choose to become couch potatoes, we do so at our own risk.

Lessons from Primitive People

Would you like to live to be 100? For years, we have heard tales of communities where centenarians are commonplace; not only that, but they are healthy and alert enough to work until they are in their eighties. Scientists and ger-ontologists (physicians who specialize in the treatment of the aged) have become particularly interested in these reports. The three regions of the world most renowned for longevity are the Ecuadorian Andes, the Karakoram mountains in Kashmir, and the Abkhazia region of the former southern Soviet Union. On-the-spot research in these areas has verified that ages of 90 to 100 years are not unusual. Heart attacks are extremely rare. Why is this so?

The inhabitants of high Ecuador and Kashmir eat sparingly of a diet low in animal fat; conversely, the Abkhazians eat well, with meat and dairy products as regular items. Smoking is common in all three areas, and most of the old people enjoy their wine, vodka, and local spirit. Researchers have remarked that in all three areas, the lifestyle is characterized by lack of stress, contentment with one's station in life, and heavy involvement of the aged in both family and civic affairs. People expect to live to a ripe old age and assume they will work for as long as they are capable. Any or all of these factors may make important contributions to their longevity. A more objective finding, however, is their high degree of cardiovascular fitness. In all three areas, their work involves heavy physical labor interspersed with a great deal of walking, not infrequently over hilly terrain. Dr. David Kakiashvili, a Russian cardiologist, is convinced that this active lifestyle, commencing in early childhood and continuing for 80 years or more, confers the high degree of cardiac health that results in such lengthy life spans. In other words, if you have a fit cardiovascular system, the odds are that you will live for a long time.

Dr. Alexander Leaf, an American cardiologist who has made a study of these people in their own environment, repeatedly found a high level of endurance fitness in the aged. He was certainly impressed with their capacity for heavy work. He wrote, "Markhti Tarkil . . . walks half a mile downhill to his daily bath in the river and then climbs uphill again. Surely any day a man can do this he must be too fit to die. The next day he repeats this physical activity and so on, day after day while the years roll by, and at 104, Tarkil is still much too fit to die!" On one occasion, Dr. Leaf toiled up a steep mountainside to interview a 106-year-old shepherd. The journey took him six hours, and the going was so rough that two of the four-man party, including the interpreter, had to turn back. The cardiologist's pride on making it to the top was, however, short-lived; it turned out that the ancient shepherd made the journey regularly in three hours! Dr. Leaf took the lesson to heart: on his return home, he commenced jogging as a hobby.

Wherever pockets of primitive peoples are still to be found, they are relatively free from heart attacks. The Kenyan Masai tribesman and the Mexican Tarahumara Indian rely mainly on their legs for locomotion. The Tarahumara call themselves the Raramuri, which literally means runner, and a ritual of their culture consists of a 100-mile (160-kilometer) foot race over rugged terrain at a seven- to eight-minute mile (four- to five-minute

kilometer) pace, at the same time kicking a small hand-
carved wooden ball! Their freedom from cardiovascular
disease is well documented.

THE EPIDEMIOLOGICAL EVIDENCE FOR THE
BENEFITS OF EXERCISE

Occupational Physical Activity

In 1953, Professor Jeremy Morris of the British Medical
Research Council published an article in the medical journal
The Lancet entitled "Coronary Heart Disease and Physical
Activity at Work." It compared the incidence of heart disease
in 31,000 male bus drivers and bus conductors working
for the London Transport Department. The drivers were
found to suffer one and a half times more anginal attacks
and twice as many fatal and non-fatal heart attacks as the
conductors. In his article, Professor Morris suggested that
the likeliest explanation for this difference might lie in the
nature of the two jobs. Driving is a sedentary activity
requiring minimal expenditure of energy; the conductor,
on the other hand, had to collect fares. In a double-decker
bus, this activity necessitates an average of 24 trips an hour
up and down the winding staircase of the moving vehicle,
in addition to walking back and forth along the aisles of
the upper and lower compartments. Over an eight-hour
shift, the energy expenditure is considerable.

Professor Morris and his colleagues were quick to point
out that this very significant association between physical
activity and immunity from heart disease was precisely that
— an association; there was no proof of cause and effect.
For instance, it might be that a process of self-selection
was at work, the coronary-prone individual being more likely
to seek employment as a driver than as a conductor.
Nevertheless, despite this very legitimate caution, the importance of Morris's pioneer work was quickly recognized.
His article was a landmark contribution, and soon other
researchers set about trying to duplicate his findings.

Israel has a high prevalence of heart disease, and its doctors have carried out much excellent research on the topic. Probably the best known to physicians is the work of Dr. Daniel Brunner. In pursuing Morris's findings, Dr. Brunner made use of a unique feature of Israeli life, the existence of the kibbutzim. In these communities, people live in a uniform environment, eating the same food, experiencing the same climate, and largely subject to the same external stresses. Obviously a study carried out in such a setting eliminates many sources of error. In analyzing the cause of death of 10,000 residents of a kibbutz over a period of 15 years, Brunner ascertained that "the incidence of angina, myocardial infarction and fatalities due to ischaemic heart disease was found to be *two and a half to four* times greater in sedentary workers than in non-sedentary workers."

In North America, work along similar lines was being carried out by the epidemiologist and physician Professor Ralph Paffenbarger of Berkeley, California. From 1951 through 1972, he studied the incidence of heart disease in some 6,000 longshoremen living in the San Francisco Bay area. This was before the advent of containerization, and he was able to stratify his subjects into light, moderate, and heavy workers. He found that the light workers had two and a half times the incidence of fatal heart attacks and three times the incidence of sudden cardiac death as did the heavy or moderate physical workers. This benefit persisted even when the ill effects of high blood pressure, obesity, previous heart disease, and cigarette smoking were taken into account. According to Paffenbarger, physical activity reduced the chance of a fatal heart attack by 54%, whereas stopping smoking or reducing high blood pressure cut the risk by only 27% and 29% respectively.

Other investigators reported similar results. Dr. Henry Taylor compared active U.S. railroad switchmen and sedentary ticket clerks; he found the latter had three times higher death rates from heart attacks. Dr. Harold Kahn, also in the United States, and Jeremy Morris in England looked at postal workers, comparing mail carriers and sorting clerks; the active carriers had one-half the heart disease of the sedentary clerks and an even greater protection against sudden cardiac death.

These are only some of the occupational studies carried out since Morris's article first appeared in 1953. With very few exceptions, they have demonstrated that people who were physically active at work had a significantly reduced incidence of death from heart disease. As for the studies that have not shown that physical work has a protective effect, the answer lies in the fact that in the jobs studied, modern technocracy has reduced the energy cost of so-called "heavy" jobs to very modest levels. As one European expert has said, "The discrepancy can be explained by the fact that nowadays work labelled as 'heavy' is not heavy at all, so that the studied population was not divided into appropriately different categories of physical activity, but rather into different categories of physical *inactivity.*"

Leisure-Time Exercise

In recent years, there has been increasing interest in off-the-job physical activity, since, as we have seen, heavy physical work has become increasingly rare. Once again, the pioneer, Professor Morris, was the first to look at this aspect of the problem. Commencing in 1968, he has examined the effect of leisure-time exercise in a group of British civil servants. In articles published in 1973, 1980, 1987, and 1990, he has demonstrated that those who reported carrying out vigorous recreational activities in their leisure time, such as brisk walking (in excess of four miles or 6.5 kilometers per hour), swimming, badminton, jogging, digging in the garden, hill walking, and other similar activities, have one-half to one-third the incidence of coronary disease of those whose recreational activities were more sedentary. This benefit persisted, even when taking into account the effect of other risk factors such as cigarette smoking, high blood pressure, diabetes, and obesity. Of course, the absence of these other risk factors heightened the benefit of physical activity. For instance, exercisers who did not smoke had about one-fifth the incidence of heart attacks as sedentary subjects who were smokers. Furthermore, the reduction in deaths from heart attacks in the exercisers was not offset by an increase in death from other causes, as was seen in the drug cholesterol trials, since *total* mortality was also lower in the exercisers. A history of engaging in vigorous athletics or team sports when young, which might indicate a genetic advantage, was not by itself associated with a lower incidence of coronary disease. "What matters," said Morris, "is the *current activity*, and compared with that the history when young is immaterial."

Professor Ralph Paffenbarger has also studied the effect of vigorous physical activity in leisure time. He followed 50,000 college alumni aged 35 to 74 years, from 1962 to 1978. During this period, those with sedentary recreational habits had 64% more heart attacks than the exercisers. Again, the charge of "preselection" is forestalled by the fact that college athletes who became sedentary in adult life showed no protective effect, while academicians who had taken up vigorous sports after leaving school did. A further refinement of this particular study was the emergence of a "threshold" of exercise at which the maximal degree of protection pertains. This worked out to be 2,000 kcal a week — or about 20 miles (32 kilometers) of walking or jogging a week (Figure 29).

Professor Paffenbarger estimated that if all the alumni had exercised, the number of heart attacks would have been reduced by 26%. If none had smoked cigarettes, heart attacks would have been reduced by about 25%. If none had been hypertensive, rates would have been reduced by about 16%. This study is equally impressive when we come to look at death from all causes, or total mortality. Here again,

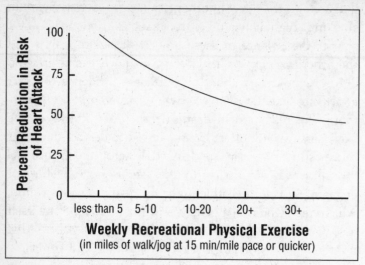

Figure 29: Exercise and Heart Attacks
The graph shows the percentage reduction of the incidence of heart attacks in Harvard University alumni according to their recreational exercise habits. The energy expended in various training activities is shown as miles of walking/jogging per week. (Source: Paffenbarger).

over the 16 years of follow-up, the physically active showed a 31% lower overall death rate than the sedentary.

A 20-year follow-up carried out by Dr. Martha Slattery and co-workers from the University of Minnesota and published in 1989 also studied the relation of leisure-time physical activity to coronary deaths and deaths from all causes. The results showed that subjects who exercised regularly had a 30% to 40% lower death rate from CHD and from all other causes compared with those who were sedentary. The amount of exercise required was equivalent to 2 miles (3 kilometers) of brisk walking, five times weekly.

Finally, you will recall the Multiple Risk Factor Intervention Trial, MRFIT, described in Chapter 4. The 12,000 men in this study were reclassified by Dr. Arthur Leon and his colleagues from the University of Minnesota according to their habitual leisure-time exercise habits and divided

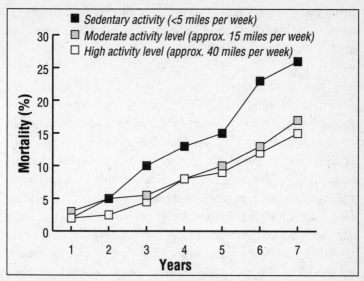

Figure 30: *Leisure-Time Physical Activity and Fatal Heart Attacks*
The graph shows that individuals who engage in moderate to high levels of exercise experience relatively lower mortality from heart attack than those who are more sedentary. (Source: Leon *et al.*)

into high-, moderate-, and low-level exercisers. The average energy (in terms of miles or kilometers walked/jogged per week) spent by the light exercisers was 5 miles (8 kilometers), the moderate 15 miles (24 kilometers), and the high 45 miles (72.5 kilometers). Over the seven years of follow-up, the high and moderate groups were found to have an increasingly lower incidence of fatal heart attacks and sudden cardiac death (Figure 30). You will note that there was no advantage in exercising above the moderate level, a similar finding to Paffenbarger's.

The evidence that physical activity protects against coronary disease is very convincing, as is the evidence that physical inactivity is a separate risk factor for heart disease, acting independently of the other known risk factors. Of course, a totally conclusive epidemiological study is impossible. It has been estimated that to provide 100% statistical proof, you would have to launch a clinical trial involving some 8,000 subjects, randomly allocate them to an exercise and a non-exercise group, and follow them up for a minimum of five years, an impossibly costly undertaking.

There is, however, another approach we can employ. The late Professor Bradford Hill, a renowned English medical statistician and pioneer in the field, devised a series of complex tests, nine in all, that could be applied to epidemiological data in order to prove its validity. At this stage, one of the best known public health institutions in the world, the Centers for Disease Control in Atlanta, Georgia, enters the picture. Workers from that prestigious organization decided to settle the exercise-heart disease question once and for all. After an extensive and systematic review of all the medical literature on the topic, they chose the 43 largest and most well-designed studies and, using Bradford Hill's criteria, subjected all of the data to a rigorous meta-analysis. The results were published in 1987. In summary, they reached the following conclusions:

1. It is proven that physical activity is inversely and causally related to the incidence of coronary heart disease. In other words, physical activity protects one from coronary disease.
2. Physical inactivity is a major coronary risk factor, equal in magnitude to hypertension, hypercholesterolemia, and cigarette smoking.
3. Public health strategies to prevent coronary heart disease should promote physical activity as vigorously as measures to reduce the other risk factors.

As if that were not enough, the authors make further pertinent observations. Looking at the other risk factors, they point out that (i) 36% of the American population are at risk for a heart attack because of hypertension, (ii) 25% to 40% are at risk from high blood cholesterol, and

(iii) 30% are smokers. On the other hand, 60% of the population are physically inactive. Obviously, removal of all four is the desirable goal, but seen from this perspective, exercise assumes its rightful importance.

Finally, after nearly 50 years of epidemiological research, and thanks to the unceasing efforts of scientists such as Morris, Paffenbarger, Brunner, and many others, the case for exercise in the primary prevention of CHD has been made. Although this simple fact seems to have become lost in the veritable welter of information about diet, fats, and cholesterol, I am confident that ultimately a more balanced approach will prevail.

The Medical Evidence for the Benefits of Exercise

One of the earliest advocates of exercise training for cardiac patients was an Irish physician, William Stokes. In his classic medical textbook, *Diseases of the Heart and Aorta*, published in 1854, he described what he called his "pedestrian cure." It consisted of slow walking on level ground, the pace to be prescribed by the physician, with undue breathlessness and chest discomfort to be avoided. As the patient's condition improved, the duration and speed of the walk was increased. Stokes reported considerable success with this method, describing how some of his patients progressed to the stage where they could easily manage brisk walking over hilly terrain. His teaching was largely forgotten until the latter part of the nineteenth century, when it was taken up again by Dr. Oertel of Munich, who combined the walking therapy with a weight-reducing diet for his heart patients.

By this time, however, a totally different philosophy to illness had evolved, and it was to bury the exercise approach for the next hundred years. In 1863 the famous London surgeon Dr. John Hilton published a book called *Rest in Pain*. In it he maintained that the most effective way to help a patient recover from an illness or a surgical procedure was to allow the body full scope to use its own natural defense mechanisms. This could be achieved only, he said, by enforcing strict bed rest. Unfortunately, his admonition was carried to the extreme. When I was a medical student, patients recovering from heart attacks bore the full brunt of this form of treatment. Immobilization was the order of the day; little, if any, movement was permitted — except the mandatory daily bowel movement. Even this was performed between the sheets, with the patient perching precariously on the ubiquitous bed pan (an endeavor, ironically, later found to be more energy consuming than using the toilet).

One of the first to take issue with the strict bed rest philosophy was Dr. William Dock, a California physician who during the 1940s published an article entitled "The Evil Sequelae of Complete Bed Rest." In it he stated bluntly that lying flat for days on end could lead to severe depression, pneumonia, blood clots in the leg veins and lungs, back problems, muscle wasting, softening of the bones, and even sudden cardiac death in heart attack patients who were struggling to use a bed pan while lying on their backs.

In the 1950s, two Harvard Medical School cardiologists, Dr. Samuel Levine and Dr. Bernard Lown, described their revolutionary "armchair" treatment. Of 73 patients admitted to hospital for a heart attack, 15 were taken out of bed and nursed in an armchair on the first day, 30 on the second, 18 on the third, and the remaining 10 on the fourth to the ninth days after their attacks. Contrary to the prevailing fears of the time, they did not suffer ruptured hearts and premature death. In fact, they all made excellent recoveries. One of the most spectacular features of the treatment was their patients' enhanced sense of well-being and relief from anxiety. The period of convalescence was shortened considerably, and there was an earlier return to work. This experiment marked the turning point in the treatment of heart attacks and led to the widespread acceptance of early mobilization during the 1960s, and eventually to the concept of exercise rehabilitation in the 1970s.

Evidence from Aerospace Medicine for the Benefits of Exercise

Many of the clues to the ill effects of prolonged bed rest came from experiments carried out on healthy volunteers, including highly trained athletes. Confinement to bed was inevitably accompanied by a marked loss of fitness, as well as severe "deconditioning" of the cardiovascular system. Valuable as this work was to medicine, it assumed even greater importance in the 1960s when man first ventured into outer space. Prolonged exposure to the weightlessness of space flight was found to produce a deconditioning effect similar to bed rest. Some of the hallmarks of the effect were a rapid pulse rate, reduction in the size of the heart and the amount of blood it ejected per beat, and a drop in blood volume and red blood cell size. The end result of these cardiovascular changes was a marked deterioration in the capacity for physical work. Add to this the development of an unstable blood pressure, softening of bones from loss of calcium in the urine, and severe muscle wasting, and you have a frightening list of disabilities. Small wonder that considerable investigation went into solving the problem of deconditioning.

Space travel gave a potent incentive to the investigation of all aspects of cardiovascular fitness. Apart from using prolonged bed rest, considerable data on the subject of fitness and deconditioning also accumulated from the early American Gemini, Apollo, and Skylab missions, as well as the Soviets' Vostak and Soyuz flights. We now know that many of the manifestations of deconditioning can be prevented by a planned exercise routine. All space flight crews are now obliged to carry out regular in-flight training regimens, using cycle ergometers and treadmills.

PHYSICAL ACTIVITY VERSUS PHYSICAL FITNESS

Although all these epidemiological studies have examined physical activity, none has measured the level of physical fitness that these activities confer. The shortage of such studies is understandable. An individual's physical habits can be ascertained from their occupation, a personal interview, and a questionnaire. Measurement of fitness, on the other hand, is a much lengthier procedure. It requires the use of equipment such as a stationary cycle or a treadmill, involves trained health professionals, and takes an hour or more of the subject's time.

Dr. Ruth Peters and her co-workers carried out fitness testing on 2,800 firefighters and law enforcement officers of Los Angeles County. They were divided into high and low fitness categories. Over a five-year follow-up period, the low fitness subjects had twice as many heart attacks as the high, even in the absence of other risk factors. When subjects who were unfit and possessed two or more of the major risk factors were compared to those who were fit and had the same combination of factors, the unfit subjects were found to have experienced six times the number of fatal and non-fatal heart attacks.

A collaborative study carried out between the universities of North Carolina and California determined the fitness level of 4,000 healthy men, aged 30 to 69 years, and divided them into four levels, or quartiles, the first quartile being the least fit and the fourth quartile the most fit. Over an eight-year follow-up, the death rate from all causes was much higher in those with the lowest level of fitness than it was in those with the highest (Figure 31). In fact, the first quartile compared with the fourth quartile had eight and a half times the death rate from all forms of cardiovascular disease, including strokes, and six and a half times the death rate from heart attacks alone. The results were found to be independent of smoking, cholesterol level, and blood pressure.

The men's fitness, or lack of it, corresponded to their reported level of exercise training and sports involvement, proving that a genetic resistance to heart disease was not

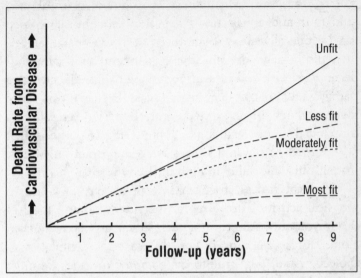

Figure 31: Death from Cardiovascular Disease According to Levels of Fitness
**Over the period of observation, the least fit individuals showed
the greatest mortality from heart attacks and strokes, while the
most fit showed the lowest mortality.** (Adapted from Ekelund *et al.*)

a factor. Also, if you look at the mortality curves in Figure
31 you will notice that they start to separate early and
continue to separate even more over the course of the study,
proving that the initial difference in fitness levels was not
due to unrecognized heart disease at the beginning of the
study. If it had been, then the greatest separation would
have occurred within the first few years. Then as the sickest
subjects died, the curves would have started to come
together. This study provides one of the most convincing
arguments for the benefit of physical fitness.

In 1989, a medical team including Dr. Ken Cooper, Dr.
Ralph Paffenbarger, and Dr. Steven Blair reported on a
study of 13,344 subjects (10,224 men and 3,120 women)
who had been fitness tested at the Cooper Aerobics Clinic
in Dallas. Over an eight-year follow-up period, the unfit,
both men and women, had eight times the death rate from
strokes and heart attacks as the most fit. Also, over this

period, three and a half times the number of unfit men and four and a half times the number of unfit women died from all causes than their fit counterparts. These benefits held good even after adjustment for serum cholesterol levels, blood pressure, smoking habits, diabetes, and family history of coronary heart disease. Even in the presence of risk factors, fitness exerted a protective effect. The authors concluded, "The results . . . support the hypothesis that a low level of physical fitness is an important risk factor for all-cause mortality in both men and women."

Physical fitness, then, has been shown to relate to physical activity. Furthermore, the fitter you are, the less likely you are to die from a heart attack and possibly even some forms of cancer. For the sake of completeness, however, and to be true to the scientific method, we must now ask ourselves the ultimate question. If fitness protects against heart disease, how does it work?

MECHANISMS BY WHICH EXERCISE TRAINING PROTECTS FROM CORONARY HEART DISEASE

Animal Studies

The hearts of wild animals are thicker-muscled and more copiously supplied with coronary blood vessels than those of their domesticated cousins (for example, wild ducks versus tame ducks or hares versus rabbits). By the same token, trained greyhounds and thoroughbred race horses have larger and more efficient hearts than the family dog or riding school hack. Rats exposed to ten weeks of swimming training develop significant increases in size and number of their coronary arteries and branches. These changes are maintained so long as the rats continue to work out, but as soon as they stop training, the coronaries begin to return to their original state. Running training has been found to be just as effective as swimming.

Exercise can even increase the size and number of coronary arteries when one or more of the coronaries has been slightly narrowed. Dr. Richard Eckstein took a group of 90 dogs and, using surgical thread, artificially narrowed their coronary arteries to give them varying severities of non-fatal heart attacks. He then divided them into two groups, one group being confined to cages and the other put on an exercise program consisting of 20 minutes of running on a treadmill, five times weekly. At the end of a six- to eight-week period, he measured blood flow through the coronary arteries and noted that the exercised dogs had compensated for their narrowed blood vessels by developing new branches, known medically as collaterals. The sedentary dogs, on the other hand, showed no such effect. Eckstein concluded that "the judicious use of early and continued physical exercise may reduce the clinical manifestations of coronary disease."

The coronary anatomy of pigs is similar to that of humans. In one experiment, a group of pigs had a coronary artery narrowed so as to simulate coronary disease. One half were then trained, and the other half were not. Then the narrowed artery was closed off completely, mimicking a heart attack. In both groups, there was an immediate development of collateral vessels, but these were twice as plentiful in the trained as in the untrained animals. In addition, the area of damage to the heart muscle of the exercised pigs was only one-quarter the size of that in non-exercised animals.

Another approach has been to measure the effect of exercise training on the ability of heart muscle damaged from a heart attack to withstand the insult of recurrence. Dogs who were exposed to a "rehabilitation" exercise training program after a heart attack successfully survived a second one, whereas the non-rehabilitated dogs all died.

Much can be learned from study of the apes and the monkeys, members of the primate family of mammals to which humans belong. Take the case of the longest living gorilla in captivity, a resident of the Philadelphia zoo. Since gorillas have the same life expectancy as a human, it was confidently felt that he would live to threescore years and ten or thereabouts. Actually, he died from a massive stroke at the age of 52. Even more disturbing, the autopsy showed that during his lifetime he had sustained a number of severe non-fatal heart attacks. Gorillas are vegetarians, and great care had been taken to provide him with the identical foodstuffs he would have enjoyed in the wild. This diet, totally free from saturated fat and cholesterol, should have protected him from coronary atherosclerosis. What had gone wrong? The answer lies in another aspect of the gorilla's lifestyle. In their natural habitat, gorillas cover large tracts of territory to forage for food. In captivity this was denied him, and it was the opinion of the zoo experts that the consequent lack of regular physical activity was the main factor contributing to his premature death from coronary heart disease. Does this mean that even the so-called ideal healthy heart diet cannot offset a life of sloth?

The work of Dr. Dieter Kramsch illustrates the other side of the coin. Over a period of four years, he fed a group of macaque monkeys a diet heavily loaded with saturated fat and cholesterol, the intent being to induce severe coronary artery disease. Half of the monkeys, however, were put on a training program consisting of one hour of running on a treadmill, three times a week. Over the four years of the study, a number of the non-exercising monkeys developed angina, as well as non-fatal and fatal heart attacks. By the end of the four years, all were found to have severe coronary artery disease. In sharp contrast, all the exercise monkeys remained in good health and at the end of the study were found, without exception, to have healthy coronary arteries, which were completely free of atherosclerosis and were, in many cases, larger in size than monkeys fed a normal diet. Not only that, but the exercisers had significantly higher blood levels of the "good" HDL-cholesterol and much lower levels of the "bad" LDL-cholesterol. What better example could there be of a good training program offering protection against a bad diet?

The Human Heart: Training Changes in Structure and Function

The human heart responds to exercise by changing in size and performance. It is nearly 100 years since the first observation was made that fit, long-distance skiers had large hearts, and the fitter and more successful the skier, the larger the heart. Subsequently, and with the increasing use of X-rays, most elite endurance athletes, such as long-distance runners, cyclists, and rowers, were also found to have cardiac enlargement. This finding led to the term "athlete's heart," meaning a heart that as a result of regular training was healthy, efficient, and powerful. Unfortunately, in later years the term came to be synonymous with a diseased heart. How could this situation arise?

Until recently, physicians equated enlarged hearts with disease since a failing heart will dilate, and thus increase in size. The heart of a hypertensive, which has worked for years against a high blood pressure, will develop enormously thickened muscular walls and will therefore also increase in size. Small wonder then that examining physicians who were used to dealing with disease rather than health were suspicious of athletes with big hearts, even though they could not find any evidence of the diseases that customarily cause the pathological enlargement.

Now that we have more sophisticated methods to observe the heart, we can better understand the exact nature of the enlargement that comes with training. Echocardiography (a form of X-ray using sound waves to picture the heart and its movements) has amply demonstrated that the ventricles of the endurance athlete's heart have a larger volume and capacity than is found in the sedentary subject. This has been particularly demonstrated in the case of long-distance runners and swimmers.

Today, few would argue the superiority of the athlete's heart. Instead, they try another tack. The enlargement, they claim, is genetic and not the result of training. A number of studies have shown this to be false. A group of healthy young men and women from the Sacramento Police Academy underwent three months of endurance training, which consisted of one hour of walking and/or running, four days a week. At the end of the training period, their hearts showed an increased volume, with ventricles that contracted more briskly and ejected more blood per beat; in other words, improvement in size and function. Similar results were reported by a group of physicians from Washington University, who also demonstrated that a period of detraining tended to reverse these beneficial changes.

One of the most characteristic results of regular exercise is a drop in the resting and exercise heart rate. This lowering is referred to medically as *bradycardia* (Greek for slow heart). It is so characteristic of fitness that if it does not occur in the individual who is on a training program, you can be sure that the subject is either not adhering faithfully to the program, or that the training regime is badly designed.

To compensate for the lower pulse rate, the heart expels more blood per beat, or expressed physiologically, a greater volume of blood per stroke. This increase in stroke volume is another characteristic of the trained heart. The bottom line is a more efficient cardiac pump.

In animals, an increase in heart size is parallelled by a proportionate increase in the diameter and number of branches of the coronary vessels, together with an increase in the capillary blood vessels that course through the substance of the heart muscle. In this way, blood supply keeps pace with demand. Does this also occur in humans? Clarence DeMar, a famous American long-distance running champion, died of cancer in his seventies; an autopsy of his heart revealed that his coronary arteries were unusually large. Although this may be the result of natural endowment, it seems more likely to have been brought about by his many years of intensive training. Large coronary arteries are a distinct advantage in that they are unlikely to be blocked by even a lifetime's deposit of fatty atheromatous material.

It should also be noted that blood flows through the coronary arteries to supply the heart muscle *between* beats (that is, during diastole). Thus, the higher the heart rate, the shorter the period of diastole. Conversely, the slower the heart rate, the greater the proportion of time spent in diastole. Fitness bradycardia, therefore, is synonymous with a lengthening of diastole and thus an increase in coronary blood flow.

As if an improved blood supply to the heart were not enough, the fit exerciser has a further advantage over his or her sedentary counterpart. Fitness brings with it a reduction in the amount of blood the heart requires. Since the slowly beating heart muscle uses oxygen more sparingly, the blood flow does not need to be vigorous. It is a case of living well within one's cardiac budget.

The beneficial changes described above go a long way toward explaining why the fit heart is a healthy heart. But even if we do not possess the exotic equipment required to measure such changes, we would still be left with the simplest and yet one of the most important observations of all — the effect of training on the heart rate. We have already seen that training reduces the resting and exercising heart rate. It has a similar effect on blood pressure. We can obtain a very accurate index of the amount of work being done by the heart at any given time by multiplying the heart rate by the blood pressure. The result of this simple mathematical calculation is known as the Rate Pressure Product (RPP). Thus, if while sitting quietly reading this book, your heart rate were found to be 72 beats per minute, and your systolic blood pressure 120 mm Hg, then the work being carried out by your heart would be represented by an RPP of 8,640 (72 × 120 = 8,640). Assuming you were to put this book down, stand up, run vigorously on the spot for a few minutes so as to bring your heart rate up to 102 beats per minute and your blood pressure up to 140 mm Hg, then you would have increased your RPP, and therefore the amount of work your heart would have been required to do, to a figure of 14,280 (102 × 140 = 14,280). Obviously, if training gives you a lower heart rate and a lower blood pressure for a given intensity of exercise, then you will have a lower RPP and the work load on your heart will be reduced. Physiologically, you would get more for your money. You will see later how this reduction in Rate Pressure Product for a given work load can have a powerful effect in relieving anginal symptoms in patients with coronary heart disease.

In addition to the benefit to the heart itself, fitness improves the cardiovascular system as a whole. The large muscles of the leg and trunk (the so-called skeletal muscles) develop a greater blood supply as a result of training. There is an increase in the size and function of the specialized cells (mitochondrial cells) that extract and utilize the oxygen from the blood. This improvement at the delivery end, as it were, of the oxygen transport chain means less effort is required at the source, that is, the pumping heart. The fact that these peripheral gains are possible and, indeed, inevitable in a good endurance training program explains why even individuals who have had very severe heart attacks can nevertheless benefit from a carefully prescribed training program.

THE EFFECT OF EXERCISE ON REDUCING CORONARY RISK FACTORS

Exercise and Cholesterol

Just over 40 years ago, an article appeared in *Science* magazine, drawing attention to the fact that not all cholesterol was bad cholesterol. Paradoxically, one form of cholesterol, HDL-cholesterol, was noted to vary inversely with the incidence of coronary disease — that is, the higher the HDL-cholesterol values, the less likely you were to have a heart attack. Oddly enough, this vital piece of information was largely ignored until the 1970s. Throughout the 1980s, evidence for this inverse relationship continued to mount from a succession of trials. How can we increase our HDL-C? Unfortunately, while reducing saturated fat in our diet will lower LDL-C, it has little effect on HDL-C. Fortunately, there is another method: ample evidence now shows that regular physical exercise will increase HDL-C levels.

In 1974, Dr. A. Lopez, Associate Professor of Medicine at the Louisiana State University Medical School, published a report describing the effects of a seven-week training program on 13 young medical students. There was a significant increase in HDL-C with training. Two years later, Dr. Peter Wood, an English biochemist now working in the Stanford University School of Medicine, reported his investigation of 41 joggers who had been jogging in excess of 15 miles (24 kilometers) a week for a year. When compared with a group of sedentary men of similar age, all the joggers had considerably higher levels of HDL-C. He remarks in his article that "these very active men exhibited a plasma lipoprotein profile resembling that of younger women, rather than that of sedentary middle-aged men." Further reports verified Dr. Wood's findings.

These studies, however, looked at healthy subjects. Can the same effect be achieved in patients suffering from coronary artery disease? The answer is decidedly affirmative. In 1979, Drs. Dan Streja and David Mymin of Manitoba entered 32 middle-aged men suffering from coronary artery disease in a 13-week walk/jog program. Although there were no significant changes in total cholesterol, HDL-C levels increased significantly, and this "occurred in the absence of variations in diet, smoking habits, adiposity, or plasma triglyceride concentrations." Three years later, a report from the Cardiology Department of Victoria Infirmary, Glasgow, Scotland, described similar benefits in 19 post-heart attack men who were randomly allocated to an exercise program and were compared with 23 controls. The trial lasted for six months, and again the exercisers showed a significant increase in HDL-C levels. The level of exercise required was quite moderate, and in fact was a variation of the Canadian Air Force 5BX Plan.

I have also had the opportunity to study the effects of a one-year distance walk/jogging program on patients referred to the Toronto Rehabilitation Centre, with similar beneficial results. Interestingly, in my experience the threshold dose of exercise needed to surpass the normal sedentary HDL-cholesterol values is 12 miles (20 kilometers) per week, very much as that found by other investigators. Furthermore, the pace, which can range from 12 to 17 minutes per mile (7 to 10 minutes per kilometer), is less critical than the distance covered.

In fact, not only the distance but the length of time the subject has been carrying out the exercise program may be important. A group of scientists from the University of Pittsburgh studied 35 active postal carriers who averaged approximately 25 miles (40 kilometers) of walking weekly over a duration of 15 to 28 years. Although keen exercisers would consider the pace to be almost leisurely, nevertheless the postal workers' HDL-C levels were significantly higher than average for the age-matched population.

All in all, a large number of studies involving runners, middle-aged joggers, marathoners, tennis players, cross-country skiers, soccer players, and heart attack survivors taking part in supervised exercise programs have given us compelling evidence that physical activity improves HDL-C levels. This high level of HDL-C may be one of the major reasons that exercisers have a lower incidence of fatal heart attacks.

Exercise and Hypertension

Some years ago, a busy cardiologist who regularly refers patients to the Toronto Rehabilitation Centre program mentioned to me that he had taken up jogging 2 to 3 miles (3 to 5 kilometers), four times weekly. Apparently he had learned from a routine physical examination that he was suffering from mild hypertension. As he put it, "It was a case of taking medication or going on an exercise program, and as far as I am concerned, there was no contest." Approximately 20% to 40% of the population of the industrialized Western countries suffer from essential hypertension, and the overwhelming majority of these are classified as mild or borderline hypertensives (that is, they have a diastolic pressure between 90 mm Hg and 104 mm Hg and/or a systolic pressure between 140 mm Hg and 159 mm Hg; see Figure 13). My cardiologist friend, therefore, is in good company. Moreover, he also realized that all the anti-hypertensive drug trials showed that the benefit conferred to mild hypertensives by drug therapy was marginal, to say the least, not to mention the ever-present shadow of possible drug side effects.

A number of the major exercise epidemiological studies have shown conclusively that the physically active are less likely to be hypertensive. Paffenbarger's active Harvard alumni had a 35% lower risk of hypertension than their lazier counterparts. As if to vindicate the decision of my cardiologist friend, a 1989 study examined the incidence of essential hypertension in physicians who were members of the American Medical Joggers' Association and who jogged 10 miles (16 kilometers) or more per week and compared them with a group of non-exercising physicians. Both groups were carefully matched for age, gender, life-style, socio-economic status, etc. It turned out that only 7% of the jogging physicians suffered from hypertension, compared with 19% in the sedentary group. Furthermore, five times the number of non-joggers were currently taking, or had taken in the past, anti-hypertensive medication.

Dr. James Hagberg has carried out a meta-analysis of 25 exercise and hypertension studies, reaching the conclusion that exercise training can play a very important role in the general treatment of mild to moderate hypertension. He finds that the average reduction in pressure is in the magnitude of −1/−8 mm Hg. Interestingly, looking at all the data, women obtain greater benefit than men, −19/−14 mm Hg, as compared with −7/−5 mm Hg. Furthermore, the benefits of exercise, although they might seem modest, are the same as those reported for reduction in obesity and greater than those for relaxation therapy, biofeedback techniques, and salt restriction. In mild hypertensives, as previously noted, the benefits are greater than those obtained by any of the major drug anti-hypertensive trials. When used in conjunction with drug treatment, exercise can help reduce dosages, or in some cases allow the physician to discontinue drug therapy entirely. As a public health measure, it has the great advantage of being effective, as cost-effective as you can get, and, properly prescribed, safe from side effects.

Exercise Training and Blood Clotting
The formation of a blood clot within a narrowed athero-sclerotic coronary artery is usually the start of a chain of events leading to a heart attack. The process is initiated

by the platelet cells, which, detecting a crack in the endothelial lining, release a substance called Thromboxane A. This narrows the artery by putting it into spasm, makes the platelets sticky, and then clumps them together so as to cover the break in the lining. If the platelets cannot cover the break completely, they call on the help of a blood protein called fibrin. Fibrin forms a mesh of sticky strands that traps red cells, platelets, and other blood components to form a blood clot. This process is known as coagulation. Just as the body has a procoagulation system, it also has its anticoagulation system, which is called into use when the clot has formed in error inside an intact artery that may have a defective lining but is not perforated and bleeding. The anticoagulant system's first line of defense is at the level of platelet clumping. The healthy endothelium produces a substance called Prostacycline, which opposes the action of Thromboxane A by dilating, or widening, the narrowed artery and dispersing the clumped platelets. In fact, if the Prostacyclin is mobilized quickly enough, Thromboxane A may not even have time to exert its effects. Once the fibrin mesh is formed, however, a second process is required to dissolve the coagulated clot. Fibrin is dissolved by another substance called tissue plasminogen activator (t-PA). t-PA is now produced synthetically and is one of a group of drugs called "clot busters." Injected into a vein within six hours of the onset of the attack, it dissolves the clot in the coronary artery and reduces the area of damage to heart muscle.

How does all this tie in with exercise training? It now appears that regular physical activity enhances our anticoagulation mechanism, or, as it is known medically, fibrinolytic activity, so that it responds more rapidly and efficiently in dissolving unwanted clots. This connection was demonstrated as long ago as 1947 in a group of 20 healthy subjects who exercised by running up and down a spiral staircase, and whose blood was found to possess increased fibrinolytic activity. Similar results were reported by Dr. Sudhakaren Menon of London, who found that the clot-dissolving property of blood was increased by 65% in 58 university students who took part in vigorous games of soccer, rugby-football, and squash.

More recently, Dr. John Stratton of the University of Washington, Seattle, has reported the results of a study in which he and his co-workers trained a group of healthy men ranging in age from 24 to 82. At the end of six months, there was a marked increase in fitness, but even more important, an increase in resting levels of tissue plasminogen activator. This is the same substance now used as a "clot buster" in the modern treatment of a heart attack. Furthermore, the greatest increases in levels of tissue plasminogen activator appeared in the older subjects, the very age group most susceptible to heart attacks. It seems that the "wonder drug" has been available in its natural form and in ample quantity all along — but only to those active enough to earn it!

Exercise and Diabetes

Non-insulin-dependent diabetes (NIDD), also known as Type II diabetes, is a major risk factor for coronary disease. Diet and weight control are the cornerstones of treatment, but in recent years there has been more interest in the beneficial effects of exercise. Athletes and those who exercise regularly are known to be less likely to develop diabetes. Dr. Rose Frisch followed 5,400 college alumni into adult life and discovered that the prevalence of diabetes was 0.6% in the former athletes, compared with 1.3% for the non-athletes, despite the fact that the family history of diabetes was the same for both groups. One epidemiological study carried out in Fiji, where more than 20% of the population suffers from diabetes, showed that NIDD was twice as common in sedentary as in active men.

Dr. Bengt Saltin from the University of Copenhagen studied a group of men with chemical diabetes, a very early stage of NIDD, (see page 57). He found them to have a much lower fitness level than a group of age-matched normals. After completing three months of training, their fitness improved by 20%, and there was a distinct improvement in their glucose tolerance. After a further nine months of training, all members of the group had developed a perfectly normal glucose tolerance.

One of the most impressive examples of the value of exercise in NIDD is contained in a report from Dr. H.K. Takekoshi of Japan. A total of 103 NIDD patients were divided into three groups, one that did not exercise, one that walked leisurely for 30 minutes daily, and one that jogged for 30 minutes daily. All adhered to the same prescribed diet. They were followed for a period of ten years. At the end of that time, the jogging group showed no progression of disease and was under very good control, with good control in the walkers, but only fair to poor control in the non-exercisers.

Exercise and Stress Control

Prolonged periods of stress — or distress, as I prefer to call it — can result in the sustained release of the "fight or flight" stress hormones, adrenaline and noradrenaline. As we have seen, these substances increase the blood pressure, the heart rate, blood fat and blood sugar levels, and make the blood platelets sticky. A single bout of exercise puts these changes to the purpose for which they were intended — physical action. You can see how regular workouts repeated four or five times weekly can help us through the stresses and strains of everyday life. Certainly I find that if I hit a bad spot in the day and can go for a jog, a cycle, or play a game of tennis, everything begins to look a lot brighter, and what seemed to be an insurmountable problem gradually assumes more manageable proportions. Problems also have a way of solving themselves during a workout, largely because they are seen in perspective. When you are exercising, your mind is capable only of a superficial, holistic type of thinking; minutiae, trivia, and detail slip into the background, leaving you with only the prominent major points to consider. You no longer miss the forest for the trees.

Scientists have recently isolated from the brain and other nervous tissue a number of naturally occurring substances called peptides, which have opium-like qualities. One of these, beta-endorphin, has been reported to increase significantly in the blood after bouts of exercise. Furthermore, it has also been shown that regular training augments this response. Evidence at the moment suggests that the exhilaration, the feeling of relaxation, and the physical gratification felt as a result of a workout are due to release of these natural opiates.

Apart from these immediate benefits, however, there are the long-term effects of training on the catecholamine (adrenaline and noradrenaline) responses to stress. Work by Dr. Howard Hartley in the 1970s showed that after a physical training program the amount of noradrenaline released in response to physical stress was significantly decreased. A similar finding was reported by Professor Hollman of Germany.

The Toronto Rehabilitation Centre had an opportunity to investigate this benefit when we became involved in a multi-center randomized trial into the effects of an exercise rehabilitation program in post-heart attack survivors. The patients were randomized to control and exercise groups. Noradrenaline responses to various levels of work on the stationary cycle were measured on entry to the program and after one year. Exercise-induced noradrenaline levels were unchanged in the control group, but were significantly reduced, by 59% ($p = 0.05$), in the exercisers.

The value of such training-induced adaptations to stress cannot be overemphasized. Exaggerated surges of adrenaline-like substances have been blamed for the formation of intra-coronary clots and for leading to heart attacks and cardiac arrest. If regular exercise can smooth out these surges, it may also protect against death from heart disease.

Exercise and Mood

Mood disorders are extremely common in our modern society. It is estimated that approximately 12% of the population of the United States suffers from depression, and about 4% from some form of anxiety neurosis. While psychotherapy, medication, and various relaxation techniques are frequently used as treatment, there is an increasing tendency also for physicians to prescribe a physical activity program. They know from practical experience that patients who exercise invariably "feel better." Is there any scientific evidence that there is a measurable improvement in mood?

There have been numerous published reports on the effects of an exercise program on depression. The early studies lacked scientific accuracy because of their poor design; they had no control group, exercise was inadequately monitored, and any beneficial effect of exercise they discovered was of dubious value. The later trials have been more sophisticated and their results more valid. A recent meta-analysis of 80 such trials has established that regular exercise is a very effective anti-depressant, superior in most cases to relaxation therapy, and often as effective as psychotherapy, and when combined with psychotherapy it enhances the improvement gained from therapy. Aerobic activities such as walking, jogging, cycling, and swimming were found to be the most frequently prescribed and most effective forms of training. The anti-depressant effect began after three or four months, and the longer the program lasted, the more pronounced the benefit. Finally, the trials that showed the largest decreases in depression with exercise were those dealing with coronary patients.

A meta-analysis of reports published between 1975 and 1991 on exercise and anxiety has been carried out recently, with almost the same conclusions as with depression. Aerobic exercise is associated with measurable reductions in anxiety. These reductions are in the same order, but unlike depression, not necessarily superior to relaxation techniques. Again, the training programs began to be effective only after three months. Also, improvement is strongly associated with the duration of the workout, which has to exceed 20 minutes.

Exercise and Obesity

Although current weight reduction regimens inevitably stress calorie reduction through diet, they would be more successful if they emphasized energy expenditure as well. It was Dr. Jean Mayer, an authority on nutrition, who discovered that he could not make experimental animals obese by simply overfeeding them; they became fat only when he restricted their activity by putting them in cages. Of course, farmers have known this for generations. When they want to fatten their livestock, they don't merely increase their feed, they also limit their movement by enclosing them in small pens.

Obesity can be looked on as the result of an imbalance between energy intake and output. One would think that the more sedentary one is, the less one would want to eat. The opposite is the case. Studies have shown that sedentary employees eat more than moderately active workers. Individuals engaged in very heavy physical labor, such as lumberjacks, have greater appetites and consume more food than moderately active individuals, but they also burn more calories and so rarely become obese. Animal experiments have shown that rats that exercise for 20-, 40-, and up to 60-minute sessions at a time tend to eat less than their sedentary counterparts. Only when the exercise sessions exceed two hours at a time does their appetite increase. In summary, it appears that there is a level of activity below which our appetite does not relate to our energy requirements. Paradoxically, the less you do, the more you eat.

When we attempt to reduce body weight by diet alone, the weight loss consists not only of fat tissue, but also non-fat tissue (muscle and water). An exercise program, on the other hand, will burn fat, but by building muscle will increase non-fat body weight. For the first two to three months of training, the fat loss will often be balanced by an increasing amount of muscle and by water that is not being lost. Your bathroom scales may show little or no weight reduction, and if you don't take these physiological facts into account, you are likely to become very discouraged; you may even stop exercising altogether. During this stage, a better indication of your progress is the fit of your clothing.

Professor Michael Pollock of the University of Gainesville, Florida, advises that to lose weight, the workouts should last for at least 30 minutes, and the frequency should not be less than three to four times weekly. These guidelines have been confirmed by other experts in nutrition who have also found that walking, jogging, and cycling are among the most effective weight-reducing activities. The 30-minute minimum is probably due to the fact that after this length of time the muscles have switched over almost entirely from sugar to fat as their source of fuel. Swimming, for some as yet unexplained reason, does not reduce weight, although it is surmised that this may have something to do with the temperature of the water.

As a treatment for obesity, exercise has another distinct advantage over dieting alone. Exercise also improves a person's mood, whereas dieting alone often leads to an increased irritability and depression. The lifestyle change is also more permanent, and the weight loss more long-lasting.

To lose weight, most of us do best on a combined program of dietary restriction and exercise. Professors Zuti and Golding compared this combined approach to dieting alone and to exercise alone. The dieters reduced their intake by 500 calories a day. The exercisers increased their energy output by 500 calories per day, exercising five times weekly. The combined therapy group reduced their intake by 250 calories daily and increased their energy expenditure by 250 calories daily. At the end of 16 weeks, individuals in all three groups had each lost approximately 12% body weight. However, the composition of that loss was quite different. The two exercise groups lost more body fat and increased their lean body mass, whereas the diet group lost less fat and also lost lean body mass (Figure 32).

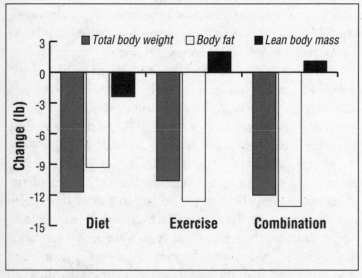

Figure 32: The Physical Effects of Dieting and Exercise
The graph shows the changes in body weight, body fat, and lean body weight brought about by dieting, regular exercise, and a combination of the two. (From W.B. Zuti and L.A. Golding)

CONCLUSION

We now have conclusive evidence that lack of physical activity is a major risk factor for heart disease and that regular exercise can play a powerful protective role. In addition to improving the pumping power and efficiency of the heart, physical training has been shown to exert a favorable influence on the other coronary risk factors. Improvement in fitness brings about beneficial changes in HDL-cholesterol and triglyceride levels, insulin sensitivity and glucose metabolism, blood-clotting mechanisms, and the levels of stress hormones. Hypertension is improved and obesity reduced. The regular exerciser feels better and is more highly motivated to adopt a healthy lifestyle and abstain from smoking and a "junk-food," high-fat diet. Finally, this healthful prescription is free; your only investment is time. All in all, I think you will agree, an impressive list of benefits.

7. Exercise Training for Heart Fitness

So far we have talked about the cardiovascular benefits of physical fitness without defining what we mean by the term. A fit sprinter can cover 100 meters in under 10 seconds, but would probably have to drop out after the first mile of a 26-mile marathon race. Obviously, there are different types of fitness.

I chose the examples of the sprinter and the marathon runner not only because they are extremes, but also because they are perfect examples of the two categories into which muscle activity and physical fitness can be divided: anaerobic and aerobic.

Working muscles use only two fuels — carbohydrate and fat — both of which burn most efficiently in the presence of oxygen. So long as there is a steady supply of oxygen from the bloodstream, muscle action will continue until all the stored fuels are used. This type of muscle action, since it utilizes oxygen, is referred to as aerobic; literally, working with air. The elite marathon runner who completes the 26-mile (42-kilometer) course in two to two and a half hours is an aerobic-type athlete. His body first runs on its stores of carbohydrate, in the form of glycogen, after which it switches to its fat stores.

When a sprinter runs at top speed, her leg muscles use a process that burns glycogen only and does so in the absence of oxygen; this process is therefore referred to as anaerobic. Unfortunately, it can continue for no more than ten seconds, after which large quantities of the by-product lactic acid build up in the muscle and slow down its contractions. Once the sprinter stops, the lactic acid has to be disposed of and the muscle fibers refreshed. This clean-up process requires oxygen. In other words, the oxygen debt built up during the ten-second sprint has to be paid back. Now you know why the sprinter, a sugar-burning anaerobic athlete, can run the entire 100 meters without taking a breath, but once past the finish line doubles over, hands on knees, gasping for air.

Of course, most athletic activities require a combination of aerobic and anaerobic effort, in varying proportions. A 400-meter run will require an equal balance of both. A cross-country ski racer will perform aerobically on the flat, but anaerobically when climbing hills. For most of the 90 minutes of a soccer game, the level of activity is aerobic, interspersed with short bursts of speed requiring anaerobic muscle contractions. Nevertheless, we can say that long-distance running, cycling, and swimming are aerobic sports, depending largely on muscle endurance, and sprinting, weightlifting, and competitive squash are predominantly anaerobic sports.

From a medical viewpoint, the distinction is very important because it is the aerobic activities, and the type of endurance fitness they confer, that lead to the cardiovascular benefits described in the previous chapter. Superior aerobic fitness is associated with an efficient oxygen transport system. The major links in this chain, you will recall, are extraction of oxygen from the air by the lungs, where it becomes attached to the hemoglobin in the blood to form oxyhemoglobin and is then pumped by the heart to the working muscles, to be transferred to a substance in the muscles called myoglobin, which shuttles it to the tiny "metabolic factories" in the muscle fibers called mitochondria, where finally the oxygen fans the flame that burns the two muscle fuels, glycogen and fat.

PRESCRIPTION FOR AEROBIC FITNESS

If a physician were to offer you a medicine that was free, had no side effects, and was guaranteed to improve your heart, blood, and muscular system, would you accept it? I think you would. You might be surprised, however, to find that the medicine came neither in a bottle, nor by injections, but was in fact a well-designed endurance-type exercise training program. If this sounds too simple, stop for a second and think of the incredibly complex changes exercise can bring about. It will (i) increase the amount of hemoglobin in your blood, (ii) improve the efficiency and blood supply of the heart while at the same time making it more resistant to coronary heart disease, (iii) add to the supply of myoglobin and network of blood vessels in the working muscles, and (iv) enhance the number and effectiveness of the muscle mitochondria so that they can burn fat more efficiently. All in all, you will agree, an imposing list of advantages.

When I prescribe a drug I specify its name, the strength of the dose, the number of times it should be administered each day, and the duration of the treatment time. Writing a prescription for exercise is no different. I have to specify the mode or type of activity to be followed, the strength or intensity with which it must be performed, the frequency of workouts, and the duration of each workout.

Of these four components, exercise intensity is the most critical, since it determines the effectiveness and safety of the training program, a particularly important consideration for middle-aged people and those with heart disease. Let's consider it in some detail.

Intensity of Workout

If you want to train for an anaerobic event like a 100-meter sprint, you have to get your muscles used to burning sugar at a prodigious rate and to performing without oxygen for short periods at peak efficiency. Therefore, your workouts must simulate these conditions; they must be carried out at very high intensity and for brief bursts. The aerobic athlete, on the other hand, needs to conserve the body's meager stores of glycogen (only one pound or 500 grams), start to burn fat (of which there is an almost unlimited supply) at an early stage of the training session, and ensure a constant supply of oxygen to the muscles. The workout should be carried out at an intensity low enough to permit it to reach the fat-burning phase, which occurs after about 20 to 30 minutes of exercise, without incurring an oxygen debt.

The intensity of the workout is thus determined by its duration. The higher the intensity, the sooner the exerciser has to quit. For instance, a novice exerciser may not be able to complete a 30-minute walk if the pace exceeds 4 mph (6.5 km/hr), or a 15-minute-mile (9-minute-kilometer) pace. On the other hand, that same exerciser might be able to walk for 30 minutes at a snail's pace of, say, 1 mph (1.6 km/hr). However, such a low level of intensity would produce little or no aerobic training effect (unless one were a snail). Nevertheless, the concept that "duration determines intensity" is a useful one and is employed to advantage in the "out and back" training method. Here, the walker or jogger who wants to complete a 30-minute workout is required to proceed from a starting point, at a steady pace, for a period of 15 minutes, and then return by the same route at the same pace. If the starting point has not been reached by the 30-minute limit, then the outgoing pace was obviously too quick; if it is reached with time to spare, then the pace was too slow.

In the days before coaches were exercise physiologists with postgraduate degrees from prestigious universities, you would often hear them exhorting their athletes to carry out a workout at "half effort," or "quarter effort" or "almost full effort." This instruction may have sounded vague to the uninitiated, but both the coach and the athlete knew what was meant. The principle was a good one and, in fact, is the basis for another approach we use today in aerobic training. The only difference is that we now measure and express effort in terms of scientific units.

Oxygen Intake

Aerobic fitness is evaluated by measuring the maximum volume of oxygen the athlete can burn. This volume is expressed in liters of oxygen per minute, or if you take into account body weight, milliliters of oxygen per kilogram of body weight per minute (mL/kg/min). This maximum is referred to as the athlete's peak oxygen intake, or aerobic power; the higher it is, the better is the athlete's chance of competing successfully in an endurance-type event. Thus, an athlete with a maximum oxygen intake (often abbreviated to VO_2max) of 80 mL/kg/min will perform better in a long race than one with a VO_2max of 50 mL/kg/min. In other words, the former has a superior oxygen transport system. Once we have established someone's VO_2max, we can convert this into a running, cycling, or swimming speed, and then take one-half or one-third of this number to give the training pace equal to the old coach's one-half or one-third effort. For example, if you have a VO_2max of 35 mL/kg/min, then this tells us that you are capable of running a mile in 10 minutes or a kilometer in 6 minutes. A training pace that calls for two-thirds effort would be one which utilized 23 mL/kg/min ($35 \times 2/3 = 23$), which is equivalent to a 12-minute-mile (7.5-minute-kilometer) pace. The same calculation can be worked out for any percentage of VO_2max and expressed in the appropriate pace of any aerobic-type sport. To improve aerobic or endurance fitness, it has been established that the training workouts should be between

40% and 80% of one's VO_2max. At the lower end of the scale will be the very unfit, or the patient with coronary disease, while at the upper end is the fit athlete.

How do we measure maximum oxygen intake? The air around us contains 21% oxygen. Analysis of the air we expire, or breathe out, will show a reduction in this percentage; the difference represents the amount of oxygen consumed by our bodies. When you are relaxed or sleeping, this amounts to 3.5 mL/kg/min. Some exercise physiologists, particularly those in North America, refer to this rate of oxygen utilization at rest as a MET, and levels of activity above resting as multiples of a MET. For example, the oxygen cost of running a 10-minute mile (6-minute kilometer) is 35 mL/kg/min, or 10 METs (10 × 3.5 mL/kg/min). The more vigorously we exercise, the harder our muscles work, the more oxygen they require. Ultimately, however, the point will be reached where the oxygen transport system can no longer cope with the muscles' increasing demands for oxygen. So far, and no further, they say. The most important limiting factor in this process — the link in the oxygen chain that determines when the body has reached its limit of oxygen utilization — is the heart. Once the heart has reached a point beyond which it cannot increase the amount of blood it pumps per minute (maximum cardiac output), then greater physical effort is impossible. This is yet another expression of the fact that the level of your aerobic fitness is an index of your heart's health.

To test a person's maximum oxygen intake, we have to carry out an exercise test, which requires trained personnel and sophisticated equipment. We use a treadmill or a stationary cycle and increase the work stages every one or two minutes until the subject has to stop because of muscle fatigue. The level of oxygen intake at which this occurs is the subject's maximum oxygen intake, or aerobic power. Exercise testing, then, is the scientific way to determine aerobic power and is used to prescribe an effective

Figure 33: The Relationship Between Heart Rate and Oxygen Intake
Heart rate and oxygen intake increase together in a linear fashion as we exercise more and more vigorously. Because maximal heart rate is reached slightly earlier than maximal oxygen intake, the relative percentages of each value are slightly different. Here we see that 60% $\dot{V}O_2$ max equals 70% of HR max.

and safe training program. Because of its complexity, however, the test is reserved for elite athletes or novice exercisers who are in the coronary-prone age group, or for those who actually have coronary heart disease.

Heart Rate
Simpler procedures involve the use of heart rates, which bear a predictable relationship to oxygen intake and therefore can be measured without the use of elaborate equipment. Since heart rate and oxygen intake increase at approximately the same rate in response to increments in effort, for most purposes we can use them more or less interchangeably. However, because the maximum heart rate is achieved slightly sooner than maximum oxygen intake, the percentages of maximum are not identical (Figure 33).

Everyone has a maximum heart rate that is related to

his or her age. A 20-year-old's maximum heart rate is about 200 beats per minute, and a 70-year-old's about 150 beats per minute. A simple way to calculate your maximum heart rate is to use the equation 220 − (age in years) = maximum heart rate. This equation is not as accurate as that obtained by an exercise test and may be out by as much as 10%, but the method is accurate enough for general use in healthy individuals who are free from coronary heart disease.

Yet another method of using heart rate to prescribe effort intensity is to take a percentage of the heart rate reserve (HRR), which is the difference between the resting and maximum heart rates. This percentage is then added to the resting heart rate to give the training rate. This method, called the Karvonen method, after its developer, has been shown to give a training heart rate which is much closer to that which occurs at *the same percentage of VO_2max* than would be obtained from simply taking a percentage of maximum heart rate. For example, to work out the HRR of 60% for a 48-year-old by the Karvonen method: 220 −48 (age) = 172 (maximum HR)−72 (resting HR) = 100 × 60% = 60 + 72 (resting HR) = 132 HRR. You will note that this method gives a training rate higher than would be obtained by simply taking 60% of maximum heart rate (172 × 60% = 103). Resting heart rate is obtained by counting the pulse rate after sitting quietly for five minutes or so, or before getting out of bed in the morning. It is customary to take two or three resting counts over the period of a few days, and then average them out.

Rating of Perceived Exertion

In the early days of the Toronto Rehabilitation Centre's cardiac program, patients frequently reported that their doctors had cautioned them against activities that were too strenuous or had told them that they could return to light work only. Such counsel, while well-meaning, was obviously too vague to be of much help. One of our tasks was to attempt to quantify work, not an easy task when you realize that what a lumberjack would consider to be light work would more than likely put his physician in hospital for a week.

In fact, it was situations such as this that led Dr. Gunnar Borg, professor of psychology in the University of Stockholm, Sweden, to devise a new way of looking at physical effort. Dr. Borg observed that injured lumberjacks who were judged on the basis of standard tests to be, say, 25% disabled often claimed that their disability was much worse than had been assessed. At first glance, one might suspect the workers of deception in order to gain additional industrial compensation benefits. However, in Borg's words, "Closer investigations seldom revealed any serious deception, but rather indicated that the patient was making a sincere effort to rate himself." This and similar observations in related fields led Borg to develop his Rating of Perceived Exertion (RPE) Scale, in which the subject's perception of effort is rated numerically from 6, which represents almost no effort at all, through 20, the point at which further effort is impossible. The perception being asked for is one of overall exertion, rather than a feeling of effort or fatigue in any single part of the body. The numerical scale evolved from the fact that the original work was done with young men whose heart rates ranged from a resting of 60 beats per minute to a maximum of 200 beats per minute, and Borg discovered that the scale values of 6 to 20, when multiplied by 10, would approximate the heart rate of these individuals at the equivalent RPE. Since the scale is now used for a wide range of age groups, this simple pulse count is no longer valid. However, in any given individual, the scale does bear a remarkably consistent relationship to oxygen intake. In recent years, Borg has introduced a new rating scale, but the principles remain the same (Figure 34). The intensity of effort required for aerobic training is in the range of 12 to 14 on the original scale (3 to 4 on the new scale) or "somewhat hard." This rate is equivalent to 60% to 80% of VO_2max, 60% to 80% of Karvonen's HRR, and

Original RPE Scale		New RPE Scale	
6		0	Nothing at all
7	Very, very light	0.5	Very, very weak
8		1	Very weak
9	Very light	2	Weak
10		3	Moderate
11	Fairly light	4	Somewhat strong
12		5	Strong
13	Somewhat hard	6	
14		7	Very strong
15	Hard	8	
16		9	
17	Very hard	10	Very, very strong
18			Maximal
19	Very, very hard		

Figure 34: Ratings of Perceived Exertion (RPE)
The original and revised, simplified RPE scales. (From G.A. Borg)

70% to 85% of maximum heart rate.

People can be taught to recognize and reproduce this perception of exertion during their training workouts. The advantage of the method is that it allows for days when the conditions are adverse, such as high winds, hilly terrain, or excessive heat. On these occasions, the pace can be slowed to the required perceived exertion rating, and both the heart rate and oxygen intake will be maintained at the usual training level. The method may not be suitable, however, for all cardiac patients; it does not take into account irregularities in heart rhythm, or the effect of certain medications, such as beta-blockers, on perception of fatigue.

TYPES OF AEROBIC EXERCISE

Training for endurance fitness involves the repetitive movement of large muscle masses. Typical examples are brisk walking, jogging, swimming, long-distance cycling, and cross-country skiing. The possibilities are endless and depend on one's ingenuity and the climate in which one lives. The more complex the training activity, the more motor skill it requires, and the fewer people who will be able to undertake it. Also, since the ability to perform a particular sport varies widely, it is difficult to prescribe the effort intensity with true accuracy.

Walking and Jogging

I have used walking and jogging in the program at the Toronto Rehabilitation Centre for nearly 25 years, and have found these activities to be an ideal application for middle-aged subjects and for those with coronary heart disease. Walking and jogging give us greater returns of endurance fitness for a smaller investment of both time and money than any other activities I know. The skill required is minimal; the technique will be described later and can be learned in a matter of minutes. Special equipment is limited to a pair of good shoes and, if you want to go first class, a sweat suit. You can walk and jog almost anywhere — through parks, along roads or sidewalks, or around neighborhood school tracks. In cold weather, you can use the local gymnasium, covered shopping malls, or even underground apartment garages (provided they are equipped with good fume-extractor fans). Opportunities are legion; the only basic requirement is motivation. I will deal with walking and jogging in greater detail in Chapter 10. Let us look now at other forms of aerobic exercise.

Outdoor Cycling

Cycling can be an excellent form of aerobic training. After all, some of the fittest aerobic athletes in the world are long-distance cycling champions. However, one needs good roads and, at least for cardiac patients, flat terrains to maintain a steady moderate intensity. In most large North

American cities, cycle paths are a rarity, the motorists reign supreme, and one has to use extreme care. In cities with climates like Toronto's, the activity is limited to the summer months, since the roads in winter are frequently ice- or snow-covered.

If you are lucky enough to have access to attractive flat countryside, cycling might be the ideal exercise for you. Remember that the cycling speed has to be about twice that of running or jogging. For example, if your customary jogging speed is 12 minutes per mile (7.5 minutes per kilometer), you should be cycling at around 10 mph (16 km/hr), or 6 minutes per mile (3.75 minutes per kilometer). An 8-minute-mile (5-minute-kilometer) runner would be required to cycle at 15 mph (24 km/hr) to expend the same amount of energy.

Swimming

At first glance swimming would seem to be the ideal aerobic training activity for the middle-aged subject, because it is non-weight bearing and spares the knees, hips, and back. However, there are some drawbacks. Not everyone has access to a pool. Also, the energy expended depends on the proficiency of the swimmer. The beginner can squander more calories and use more oxygen thrashing from poolside to poolside than an experienced swimmer will use completing two smooth lengths. If heart rate is used to monitor effort intensity, then it should be noted that the training rate should be 10 to 12 beats lower than used for upright exercise, and the distance should be only one-quarter of the dry land distance. For example, a 2-mile (3-kilometer) jogger whose training heart rate is 120 beats per minute would get an equivalent workout by swimming half a mile (about three-quarters of a kilometer) at a training heart rate of 110 beats per minute. The explanation for the lower training heart rate has to do with the body's horizontal position. Also, since the heart does not have to work against gravity, swimming does not provide quite as effective a training effect as in upright exercise.

For patients with coronary heart disease, the temperature of the water is quite important. Most community pools are kept at 80°–84°F (26°–29°C). Cooler temperatures can cause angina or troublesome irregularities in heart rate. In older hypertensive patients, higher temperatures can be fatiguing and can sometimes cause fainting. Needless to say, high-risk patients who might be susceptible to cardiac arrest should be discouraged from using the pool.

Cross-Country Skiing

Long a popular sport in the Scandinavian countries, this activity uses both upper and lower limbs and produces highly fit aerobic athletes. One major study has also shown that regular practitioners live seven years longer than their sedentary counterparts. The intensity of effort required can be high, with a skier who covers the ground at 5 mph (8 km/hr) using about as much energy as an 8-minute-mile (5-minute-kilometer) runner. Skiing, however, is highly seasonal, and the conditions can vary considerably, from ice through loose to packed snow. Air temperatures may also be a problem for cardiac patients. Nevertheless, fun cross-country skiing is gaining in popularity and becoming more and more a family event. Downhill skiing, incidentally, is not an aerobic activity and throws considerable isometric strain on the thigh muscles.

Stationary Cycling

The higher-priced exercycles are impressive pieces of machinery, full of bells and whistles. Some monitor your heart rate, indicate when you are in the training range, simulate cycling up and down hills, advise you as to how many calories you have burned, etc. The only essential quality, however, is an easy and accurate calibration that will reproduce the desired pedal resistance, or work load, from workout to workout, day after day. It is this feature that separates a cycle ergometer (cycle work measurer) from just any stationary exercycle. Nowadays, a perfectly adequate ergometer can be bought for about $400 to $500. Probably their greatest advantage is that they can be used indoors, leaving the exerciser with no excuse for not exercising during the extreme temperatures of winter and summer.

My experience using cycle ergometers for home exercise training programs, however, has been disappointing. I have only known one individual, a highly motivated plastic surgeon, who has used an exercycle regularly, five days a week, for a number of years. In general, most patients are enthusiastic for the first six months or so, but within a year the exercycle invariably finds it way from the study, to the bedroom, to the basement, where it eventually gathers dust for another year before it is sold to another enthusiastic neophyte exerciser. The first hint of its ultimate fate comes when the patient stations it in front of a television set so as to watch a favorite program, or tries to set up some form of music-stand arrangement that allows a book to be read while cycling. Herein, of course, lies the crux of the problem. The exercycle is too convenient. The walker or jogger has to make time in the week to leave the home or office, and maybe change and shower. The day must be planned to include the workout, and this requires a change of lifestyle. The stationary cyclist *adds* the workout to the day's activities, whether to reading or to watching television. By doing so, the cyclist admits that exercising is an option, a luxury, and not an essential that has to take precedence over some other activity. Of course, if the cycling is carried out in a health club, then this situation does not apply. Not only is there the need to allow time for the visit, but there is also the companionship of fellow exercisers.

Solitary stationary cycling is incredibly boring. There is no passing scene to gaze upon, no fresh air to breathe, no variation in terrain, no wind, no rain, no sun — no fun. So, if you choose this route for your exercise program, don't invest too much money at the start. If after a year or so you are still in the saddle, then treat yourself to a luxury model.

Motorized Treadmills

Treadmills are yet another alternative. They can be expensive, $5,000 and up. Cheaper ones can be noisy, and if you weigh 200 pounds (90 kilograms) or more, you will need one with a powerful motor, and that can increase the cost. The walking or jogging action, however, is quite natural, and you can adjust the grade to simulate hill walking.

Rowing Machines

These machines are becoming more popular. They are a bit more expensive than a cycle ergometer and can provide a very strenuous workout. The semi-lying position adopted when rowing, as well as the heavy armwork required, puts more stress on the cardiovascular system than cycling. Heart rates and blood pressures are higher for a given oxygen intake. So, if you are a beginner, middle-aged, or have a history of cardiac disease, I would be cautious before investing.

Walking with Hand-held Weights

This activity, which has become popular in the past few years, is intended to increase the oxygen intake, or intensity, of a walking prescription without having to increase the pace of the walk. Let us take an example. You have a VO_2max of 32 mL/kg/min. Your exercise training prescription calls for a workout intensity of 50% of your VO_2max, or 16 mL/kg/min, which works out to a walking pace of 4 mph (6.5 km/hr), or 15 minutes per mile (9 minutes per kilometer). After you walk at this pace regularly for a while, your VO_2max improves to 40 mL/kg/min. To continue to train at 50% of your new VO_2max (i.e., 20 mL/kg/min), your pace will have to increase to 4.5 mph (7.2 km/hr), or 13.5 minutes per mile (8.5 minutes per kilometer). However, this pace would require you to jog a portion of the workout, and it may be that for some reason, say a knee or a back problem, you cannot do this. Adding 3-pound (1- to 1.5-kilogram) weights to each hand will increase the oxygen cost of the 4-mph (6.5-km/hr) walk by one MET, or 3.5 mL/kg/min, to 19.5 mL/kg/min, which is approximately the same as walking and jogging at a 13.5-minute-mile (8.5-minute-kilometer) pace. It should be noted, however, that merely carrying the weights will increase energy cost only slightly. You have to swing your arms, with elbows bent, and bring your hands up to shoulder height. For some, this parade-ground style feels unnatural and is embarrassing. It may also aggravate shoulder or elbow bursitis. More importantly, the arm work causes a disproportionate increase in blood pressure and heart rate, which may be a disadvantage for some cardiac patients. Weights heavier than 3 pounds (1.5 kilograms) will likely increase the chance of injury. I tend to prefer a natural walking or slow jogging action, but there is no doubt that for some the "heavy hands" approach has its place.

Rope Skipping

This activity was popular in the mid-1980s when it was proclaimed as one of the best ways to develop cardiovascular fitness. Since the skipping rope is easy to pack, and the activity requires little or no space, it seems ideal for business travelers and vacationers who want to keep up an exercise program while away from home. Unfortunately, for middle-aged adults who are unfit to start with, it has serious disadvantages. Apart from the fact that the technique takes some practice to perfect, it puts considerable strain on the lower legs, particularly the knees and calves. The most serious problem, however, is that it is impossible to carry out at a low intensity, which is where most of us want to start our fitness program. If you can't jog at a 10- to 12-minute-mile (6- to 7.5-minute-kilometer) pace, then you will not be able to skip for the 20 to 30 minutes required for aerobic training. In short, if you already have a good level of aerobic fitness and have learned the skipping technique, skipping is a good way to maintain your fitness while on the road. I do not advocate it for cardiac patients.

Aerobic Dancing, Dancercise

Popularized on television, video tape, and now part of every "Y" exercise menu, these continuous calisthenic activities are carried out to fast-tempo disco-type or rock music and are usually very strenuous. Unless they are specially geared to the middle-aged, sedentary person, you should not participate unless you are very fit. The potential for leg injuries is also high, although the introduction of so-called low-impact aerobics has reduced this risk somewhat. I do not recommend this type of training regimen for my cardiac patients.

Stair-Climbing Machines

These machines were introduced into fitness clubs in the 1980s. They are a modern version of stair stepping, except that they use two steps, which ascend and descend in response to the climbing action of the exerciser. The intensity of the workout can be modified by adjusting the speed of stepping and by changing the resistance required to depress the steps. Sophisticated versions include a computer program that varies the frequency and resistance of stepping to suit the weight and fitness of the subject. More recent models also include bars for hand gripping, which reproduce a climbing action.

The concept here is good, in that the intention is to use all the muscles of the upper and lower limbs for training. We have used the machines in the TRC program on a trial basis, but have found that they demand a higher intensity of effort than is suitable for cardiac patients. The energy required is often higher than the computerized program recommends, and the strain on the thigh muscles can often be greater than that imposed by stationary cycling. At this point, therefore, we do not advocate them for heart patients, although they are probably suitable for healthy young individuals looking for a compact indoor appliance to help improve their endurance fitness. I have no doubt that further refinements will result in a version more suitable for the older and less fit cardiac patient.

Step Aerobics
They say there is nothing new under the sun, and certainly this latest vogue in exercise equipment is an example of this adage. Bench stepping has been used to measure cardiovascular fitness since the 1920s. The current products on the market generally consist of a bench, about 4 feet (1 meter) long and 1 foot (30 centimeters) wide, which can be adjusted for height from about 6 up to 12 inches (15 to 30 centimeters). The exerciser steps up and down to a count of four. Intensity of effort can be adapted to suit the individual by regulating both step height and rate of stepping. It has been calculated that at 80 steps per minute the subject is using the same amount of oxygen as if jogging at a 10-minute-mile (6-minute-kilometer) pace. A cadence of 120 steps per minute equals an 8.5-minute-mile (5-minute-kilometer) pace. Advocates of this system maintain that there is less impact than jogging, although when I tried it myself I found it hard on the knees (an age-related problem, no doubt). By pumping the arms and adding weights, you can increase the intensity further. Again, there is the question of boredom. How many of us, I wonder, can adhere to a program of 45 minutes stepping, five times weekly, year-in, year-out?

DURATION AND FREQUENCY

There are two other components to be considered when prescribing a training program: the length of the training session, and the number of times it should be carried out per week. As we have seen, the duration of the workout should be at least 30 minutes, and the goal should be 45- to 60-minute sessions. More intense levels of activity may achieve the same training effect with shorter sessions, but the sedentary, middle-aged individual, or the patient with coronary heart disease, is better to make haste slowly. There is also the matter of weight reduction. Glycogen stores begin to drop after about 10 minutes of exercise. By 30 minutes, glycogen provides no more than half the energy required, and from then on the body begins to draw more and more on its fat stores. Have you ever seen an obese long-distance runner? You probably never will. The training sessions are so long that all excess fat is burned, with the result that long-distance runners have the lowest percentage body fat of all athletes. It is duration rather than intensity that burns calories. The name of the game, then, is long slow distance, or LSD.

As for the frequency of training, four to five times a week seems ideal. Nowadays, competitive athletes train seven days a week, and sometimes twice a day. Such excessive measures may well pay off when only yards or meters and seconds separate the world's best and the third-rater, but the added 1% to 2% improvement that seven-day-a-week training gives hardly makes it worth the effort for the average person. On the other hand, individuals who train less than twice a week make minimal progress. In terms of fitness payoff for time invested, four to five times a week seems to be the answer.

8. The Cardiac Rehabilitation Program

"There is no way you can go back to your old job," said the physician.

Bill H., a 39-year-old construction worker, stared across the desk in disbelief. "What can I do?" he said. "I don't know any other trade. How will I get by?"

Firmly, the doctor reminded him of the facts. Bill had just been discharged from hospital after his second serious heart attack. The first was a year ago. Bill's father had died at the age of 42 from a heart attack. One older brother had died, also in his forties, from a heart attack, and another brother had sustained a heart attack at age 38.

It was essential, said the doctor, that Bill take all sensible precautions to see that he had recovered completely before returning to heavy physical labor. His wife would have to go out to work, and he would have to stay at home to look after their two children, prepare their meals, and carry out the routine housework. This approach was hard for Bill to take, yet his common sense told him that his doctor was right; he was not in shape to withstand the physical strain of his job.

As the months went by, Bill became more and more morose. Never what you would call an abstainer, he began to drink heavily. Instead of benefiting from the enforced rest from work, his health became worse. He began to notice chest pains, some of which he thought were angina and others he thought were nerves. He was irritable with the children and downright unpleasant to his wife. Fortunately, his doctor was astute enough to realize that things weren't working out the way he had hoped. The doctor still felt that return to work was not the answer; neither was sitting at home all day.

"The less I do, the flabbier I get," said Bill, plaintively. "At this rate, I'll never work again."

Doctor and patient gazed speculatively at one another, each trying to find a solution.

Then Bill had a thought. "Why not send me to one of the Y's fitness classes? Wouldn't that build up my strength again?" As he spoke, his voice became more enthusiastic. Already he was seeing himself active and vigorous again, participating in the games and sports he had enjoyed at school.

The physician was torn. There was no doubt a fitness program would boost Bill's morale, but what of the safety factor? How could he entrust Bill and his damaged heart to a fitness class geared to the needs of essentially healthy individuals? Then, a thought stirred in his mind. Hadn't he read somewhere recently that a local rehabilitation centre had just started a postcoronary rehabilitation program? He promised Bill he would enquire further and let him know the outcome the next day.

The doctor was true to his word, and the following week, Bill was waiting in the lobby of the Toronto Rehabilitation Centre. It was 1968, and he was one of the first patients referred to the new exercise rehabilitation program for heart attack patients.

Stuart K. was 54 years old. He had "had it with doctors." And his doctors had almost "had it" with him. A highly successful executive, Stuart was a prime example of the uncooperative patient. He had just been discharged from hospital after recovery from his second heart attack. The first was only three months earlier, and his reaction at that time had been truly macho — hang tough and stay in there fighting. In Stuart's terms, this meant denying that he was suffering from anything other than a minor setback. He discharged himself from hospital one week earlier than his cardiologist advised and returned to work the following week. Shortly after this, he put himself on an exercise training program as outlined in a popular book on fitness.

Since he considered himself a rather fit individual, he skipped through the precautionary chapters of the book, and started halfway up the training table at a level suitable for those whose fitness rating was good.

In short, Stuart did all the wrong things. Small wonder that six weeks later, while on a business trip and shortly after attempting a 7-minute-mile (4-minute-kilometer) run through Stanley Park in Vancouver, he experienced severe chest pain. On his return to Toronto, he was diagnosed as having sustained another, and this time more extensive, heart attack. He was lucky enough to survive, and one would have thought that after that experience he would have adopted a more cautious approach. Obviously, caution was not his nature; if nothing else, one has to give him an A for persistence. He was still determined to work, worry, and play at his customary pre-attack level.

He presented his hapless cardiologist with an ultimatum: "Tell me how to get fit and strong again, or send me to someone who can."

His physician, feeling that Stuart had had a great deal more luck than he deserved and anxious to protect him from further excesses, recalled reading of an exercise rehabilitation program being carried on in the city. He recommended the program to Stuart.

"My God," said Stuart. "Rehabilitation! You mean basket weaving?"

"Not quite," said his doctor.

The rehabilitation program to which these men were referred was unique in that it stressed prolonged endurance exercise. If Stuart expected basket weaving, he was in for a shock. From the outset each participant would be asked to walk for half an hour, at a pace based on performance on an initial exercise test, five times a week. Within a matter of weeks, the time would be increased to one hour. The ultimate goal would be four miles (6.5 kilometers), five times weekly.

The starting level and rate of progression would depend upon the results of rigorous cardiorespiratory fitness testing. The exercise plan would be carefully tailored to accommodate each person's two-fold need: developing endurance fitness, and doing so with minimal risk to an already damaged heart. The individual would be given a prescription specifying duration, intensity, and frequency of exercise.

All patients would be expected to attend exercise classes regularly until they achieved their fitness potential. During these supervised sessions, they would be observed by physicians, therapists, and physical educators to see how they performed. If they developed cardiac symptoms, they would be examined again or their electrocardiogram would be monitored while they exercised. They were all instructed in the art of taking their own pulse, reading a stop watch, pacing themselves, and jogging in an easy and relaxed manner so as to avoid minor injuries to muscles, tendons, and joints.

Physician-led discussions would deal not only with the physiological and medical aspects of endurance training, but also the significance of exercise-induced symptoms associated with coronary heart disease. Individual advice on whether to participate in other sports such as squash, weight lifting, tennis, or curling would be available.

Bill, Stuart, and the others were going to discover that many of the sports in which they had taken part, under the impression that they were good for their health, were actually of little value in attaining true worthwhile fitness; and that a set of singles tennis played on odd occasions through the year to a perspiring, gasping, knee-trembling finish did more harm than good. But more important, they were going to find that they were expected to work constantly and assiduously on their own, changing their lifestyle to accommodate five sessions of exercise every week. Their reward? Something that money cannot buy. They would experience the sheer physical elation of being fit.

The Origins of the Program

How did the program at the Toronto Rehabilitation Centre get started? The remarkable escalation in the incidence of heart attacks, together with the realization that the survivors were still in peril from a fatal recurrence, led me in 1967 to realize that something more than routine follow-up by a physician was required. If all the risk factors were to be covered, a change in lifestyle was required. Granted, such risk factors as high blood pressure, diabetes, and high blood levels of cholesterol can be controlled by regular visits to the physician, but matters such as physical activity, diet, stress, and giving up smoking require more prolonged attention, help, and advice.

Most sedentary workers can increase their physical activity only by an exercise program carried out in their non-working hours. To obtain advice from the physician on such a program is, as many patients will attest, notoriously difficult. The plain fact is that most physicians have not been trained to prescribe exercise.

As a result of Levine and Lown's introduction of their armchair treatment for heart attack patients, it gradually became the accepted practice to mobilize these patients at an earlier stage. Then, by the 1960s, pioneers such as Dr. Hermann Hellerstein of Cleveland, Dr. John Naughton, then of the University of Oklahoma and now Dean of Medicine at the University of Buffalo, New York, and Dr. Peter Rechnitzer of Western University, Canada, were reporting successful results with postcoronary patients entered into walking and calisthenic programs. Further afield, Dr. Brunner of Israel compared a group of 64 patients in his exercise program with another group of 65 postcoronary patients who had not followed any exercise regime. Over the period of a year, there were four recurrences and two deaths in the exercise group; the non-active group had nine recurrences and seven fatalities. Dr. Victor Gottheiner, also from Israel, published a most comprehensive report of his experience in exercising 1,100 patients with coronary heart disease. Using a variety of endurance activities such as brisk walking, jogging, cycling, swimming, and rowing, he was able to demonstrate that his methods were both safe and effective.

How the Program Operates

In 1967, I drew up plans to introduce the TRC Postcoronary Exercise Program. The aim was to offer positive advice and help and to instill a pattern of healthy lifestyle habits. The main component would be exercise, around which would be built the educational aspects.

The type of exercise chosen was walking, progressing where appropriate to jogging. For patients who had difficulty walking, we used stationary cycles and swimming. In recent years, we have also added strength training with light weights for patients who need to improve their upper body strength or those who suffer from extreme muscle weakness. Walking and jogging still remain our favourite forms of aerobic training. They require little in the way of equipment or expensive facilities; their intensity, duration, and frequency can be controlled, and they are excellent builders of endurance fitness.

Postcoronary exercise programs are plagued by poor attendance and high drop-out rates. After the first flush of enthusiasm, the exerciser finds that regular attendance disrupts his or her social or business commitments. This problem is worse in a large city, where one often has to travel long distances on traffic-clogged roads and highways. The answer is to reduce the number of weekly medically supervised sessions to the minimum and have patients work out on their own the rest of the week. After all, if one cannot be taught to exercise prudently when away from the watchful eye of the physician, how can one be expected to cope with the inevitable sudden physical stresses and strains of normal everyday living? Also, if safe exercise rehabilitation programs are to become universally available, the logistics of the situation make it mandatory that medical staff be used for the maximum good of the maximum number; physicians, nurses, and therapists are in short supply, and their services should be deployed carefully.

We decided, therefore, that patients would exercise as a group at the Centre under medical supervision only once a week. Since a greater frequency of training is needed for attainment of endurance fitness, four additional home workouts would also be required. This approach has worked very well. Our patients have become fit and attend the weekly session with great regularity; indeed, the program has one of the lowest drop-out rates recorded.

All patients must be referred by a physician. The referral documents, together with hospital reports and electrocardiograms, are carefully studied by the Centre's doctors to see if there are any reasons not to exercise. The patient is then brought to the Centre for a complete examination. His or her height, weight, muscle power, and percent body fat are recorded, together with a routine electrocardiogram. Finally, the patient performs a maximal exercise test, either on the cycle ergometer or on the treadmill. A walking/

jogging exercise plan is now prescribed on the basis of the test results. The prescription states the specific distance to be covered and the time it should take. It calls for five workouts a week, one of which is carried out under supervision.

Repeated exercise tests show whether there is any improvement in fitness; if there is, a new program is prescribed. In this way, the patient progresses safely and at a rate based on his or her increasing level of fitness.

All patients are required to keep an exercise log that they hand in every two weeks. This log records their current prescription, the distance and time of each workout, and their pre- and postworkout heart rates. It also has space for noting any adverse symptoms experienced during a particular workout. The logs are read carefully by the treatment staff, and the distances, times, and heart rates are carefully charted for each patient. In this way, progress can be easily gauged at a glance. Adverse symptoms are underlined in red and immediately passed through to the physician for his or her attention. If necessary, the physician will phone the patient to clarify some remark or even to suggest that the exercise pace be reduced, or exercise training be stopped, until the next supervised session.

Traditionally, isometric training has been excluded from the cardiac patient's program, for what are good physiological reasons. A static muscle contraction that involves 75% or more of maximum effort shuts off the blood supply to that muscle and results in a compensatory increase in heart rate and blood pressure. This could be potentially harmful to the ischaemic heart. However, in recent years, there has been increasing interest in this form of training, using new types of weight-training equipment. There are also indications that cardiac patients may undertake *supervised* and *prescribed* weight-training programs without risk, provided that the weights are relatively low in respect to maximal effort (usually no more than 50% of full effort), and that they are capable of being lifted ten times in succession without excessive strain. Care should also be taken to avoid breath holding (Valsalva maneuver).

A good use for light weight-training is in preparation for return to an occupation that involves considerable arm work, or where the individual wants to take part in throwing or racquet sports. However, at this point in time, it seems prudent to restrict such activities to low-risk patients, at least until we have the benefit of more information.

Our studies have shown that the patient often experiences a great improvement in mood and morale within weeks of starting the program. Nevertheless, a period of at least a year is required for more objective physiological benefits to appear. When they have reached a satisfactory level, patients are "promoted" to a group that attends the Centre only once every fourth week, and still later to another group that attends only every other month. These "postgraduates" are still expected to complete and return their exercise logs every two weeks, however, and these are reviewed as assiduously as those from the weekly attenders.

Due to the steady demand from out-of-town physicians, we have also instituted an Outreach Program. The patient travels in to the Centre for testing, is instructed in the performance of the exercise prescription, and reports his or her progress by means of mailed-in exercise logs. Progressively heavier training workouts are prescribed as the patient gets fitter, returning for re-testing at three-, six-, and twelve-monthly intervals.

This book represents the final extension of the program. It is an attempt to reach individuals who are coronary-prone, or who have coronary heart disease and want to start an exercise program but lack expert guidance. Obviously, no book will substitute for personal supervision and contact, but I hope this one will help you avoid at least some of the more dangerous pitfalls.

Women in the Program

The number of women referred to the TRC program has steadily increased over the years. Nevertheless, women still constitute only about 10% of our current patient caseload. Other programs report the same proportion. This low number is due only partly to the lower incidence of heart disease in women. After all, the proportion of women to men in the coronary population as a whole is certainly in excess of 10%. Another reason might be that attendance at the rehabilitation classes could be more of an inconvenience for the housewife or a working woman with household responsibilities — or, probably more likely, an inconvenience for her spouse! It is also possible that the woman herself, or her medical adviser, or both, feel that rehabilitation is unnecessary, or is unlikely to be of help.

Nothing could be further from the truth. Actually, the woman who has had a heart attack or undergone coronary artery bypass graft surgery is often more incapacitated from angina, depression, anxiety, and poor physical conditioning than her male counterpart. If she had a job before her illness or surgery, she is less likely to go back to it. As a housewife, she often still has difficulty with physical tasks around the home. Women gain equal benefit. They improve their cardiovascular fitness to the same extent, as measured by increase in maximal oxygen intake and performance on the exercise test, thus their mood improves, their physical capacity for work increases, their obesity is reduced, and their cholesterol levels normalize. Of course, as it does for the men, the benefits depend on the extent to which they adhere to the program.

Women referred to the Toronto program are treated exactly the same as men. They use the same training tables, with the same age division and precautions. There is no earthly reason why a woman shouldn't progress to the 4-mile (6.5-kilometer) distance and even to the marathon if she is prepared to devote the time. I recall when the TRC

Joggers were out on a training run many years ago, we first met a middle-aged woman proceeding leisurely along the same track. Our next encounter was when we watched her finish a determined and gallant last in her first full marathon race. Today, at 71, Judith Kazdan has 34 completed marathons to her credit. She runs mostly on her own in training, occasionally with her husband.

A Home Program

Over the years, the two most common questions asked of me by patients and their physicians who cannot attend a supervised exercise program are: what is a safe starting level of exercise, and how does one safely increase this to improve the training effect? Obviously, there is no single answer to either question. The starting level will vary with the individual, depending upon initial state of fitness, the severity of the heart attack, age, and the presence or absence of symptoms. Any increase in the training prescription will depend upon training response, expressed subjectively in feelings of well-being, and objectively in heart rate response to the workout and to repeated stress tests. However, over the years, we have learned to streamline our exercise-prescribing technique and have developed a series of tables especially designed for heart patients. These, together with a set of progressing nomograms, should provide safe and effective guidelines for the intelligent layperson. Used with the accompanying remarks on training techniques, they constitute a home version of the Centre's program.

WHAT TYPES OF PATIENTS SHOULD BE REFERRED FOR EXERCISE REHABILITATION?

Now let's look at what particular groups can benefit from cardiac exercise rehabilitation.

After a Heart Attack

Historically, cardiac rehabilitation has been specifically aimed at people who have had a heart attack, and these patients still constitute the majority of referrals to an exercise program. However, with the advent of techniques to improve blood supply to the heart muscle such as bypass surgery, angioplasty, and atherectomy, additional groups of patients have been added.

Many post-heart attack patients make uncomplicated recoveries and do not require additional procedures. They are referred to a rehabilitation program because they or their physicians recognize the need. Some require help to return to heavy labor or to vigorous recreational activity. In others, restoration of self-confidence is needed to attain full recovery. I believe that all low-risk patients should at least be assessed for rehabilitation, and preferably by the rehabilitation team. Coronary atherosclerosis is a progressive disease, and my experience is that most will benefit from a program of risk factor reduction and physical conditioning. Even patients who consider themselves fit may be exercising at an inappropriately high intensity and would benefit from a more structured program.

A small group of survivors, approximately 20%, will have sustained more severe damage to heart muscle and will be unsuitable for, or may have refused, surgery. As we have seen for some of these people, exercise training is absolutely contraindicated. The rest need not be excluded from a good rehabilitation program. They will need varying degrees of close observation during exercise, even one-on-one supervision. The starting level of training may be low and progression slow; but attendance at the program can raise morale and vastly improve the quality of life.

Bypass Patients

In May 1967, Dr. René Favaloro carried out the first coronary artery bypass graft (CABG) procedure on a patient suffering from severe coronary atherosclerosis. Since then, the pop-

Figure 35: Coronary Bypass Surgery
A vein and an internal mammary artery graft.

ularity of the procedure has increased dramatically world-wide until it is now a commonplace operation carried out in all the major medical centers throughout the world.

Although technically complex, the operation is simple in concept. Using a length of vein from the patient's thigh, or a segment of artery taken from the chest wall (the internal mammary artery), the surgeon bypasses the atherosclerotic narrowing in the coronary artery by stitching (i.e., grafting) one end of the vein or artery onto the base of the aorta and the other into the portion of coronary artery beyond the narrowing (Figure 35).

Broadly speaking, the benefits of coronary artery bypass graft surgery can be two-fold: first, an alleviation or abolition of anginal symptoms; and secondly, an improved life expectancy, at least in certain cases. Is CABG surgery a quick cure-all for coronary artery disease? Only the most naive would come to that conclusion. First of all, there is a risk. Granted it is small, but no surgeon will give you a 100% guarantee that the result will be exactly as you wish. Also, remember that coronary atherosclerosis is a metabolic disease. Fixing the plumbing will not eliminate the cause nor indeed prevent progression of the disease process. This was brought home dramatically by a report from the Montreal Heart Institute in 1984 of a ten-year follow-up of patients who had undergone CABG surgery. Coronary angiography at the end of that period showed that 29% of the bypass grafts had blocked as a result of atherosclerosis, 33% showed atherosclerotic narrowing, and, even more disturbing, 47% of the previously healthy arteries now showed atherosclerotic narrowing. Admittedly, surgical techniques have improved considerably since then, and there is now more frequent use as a graft of the internal mammary artery, a blood vessel located in the muscles of the chest wall that is apparently very resistant to the development of atherosclerosis.

As bypass surgery has become more common, so the number of such cases referred to the TRC program has increased, until now at the time of writing they constitute about 35% of the total. Surely there can be no better expression of the way in which exercise rehabilitation has been accepted as being complementary to medical and surgical treatment of heart disease.

Coronary artery bypass surgery is a more dangerous procedure for women than men. The operative mortality rate is twice as high, 4% compared with 2%. This could be due to the fact that the female patient is older. The operation is also more technically difficult in a woman, because of her smaller coronary arteries. Then again, these results may be biased by preselection. After all, if cardiologists carry out angiography only on those women with the most severe symptoms, then those who undergo surgery are bound to have more extensive coronary disease than their male counterparts and obtain a less successful result. This might also explain why women have less relief of angina after surgery than men and continue to complain more of fatigue and physical incapacity. Nevertheless, once through the operation, their long-term five- and ten-year survival rates appear to be the same as men's.

I have always believed that for a person to gain the full benefits of CABG surgery, the patient should receive advice after surgery on exercise and lifestyle change. Unless the risk factors associated with the presence of the disease in the first place are effectively removed, then it is not surprising that some patients develop symptoms again. In our experience, the patient who adheres to the precepts of the rehabilitation program has a better long-term surgical result. Other programs similar to ours have had the same experience. Indeed, one group of Japanese investigators found that exercise prior to surgery and continued to three months afterwards significantly improved the chances of the graft remaining open thereafter.

PTCA Patients

Since 1977, there has been an alternative procedure to bypass surgery for certain potential surgical candidates. In that year, Dr. Andreas Gruentzig of Zurich performed the first percutaneous transluminal coronary angioplasty (PTCA). A thin catheter, with a distensible balloon at its tip, is inserted into the coronary artery until it reaches the narrowed area. The balloon is then inflated, so as to flatten the atherosclerotic deposit and thus restore normal blood flow (Figure 36). Compared with surgery, PTCA is a relatively minor procedure, not unlike a routine coronary angiogram. There is no surgical scar; the patient is in hospital only for a few nights and can resume normal activities in two or three days. Most major medical centers now perform the procedure. As with surgery, the major indication for PTCA is severe angina of effort, which is not amenable to routine medical treatment and drugs.

Inflating sausage-shaped balloon
Guide wire
Catheter

A *Atherosclerotic plaque
in coronary artery*

B *Dilating catheter is passed
beyond narrowed segment of artery*

C *Balloon inflated, flattening plaque*

D *Catheter withdrawn,
with reduction in size
of plaque*

Figure 36: Percutanous Transluminal Coronary Angioplasty (PTCA)

Currently, some 25% to 30% of angioplasties fail within 6 months, the atherosclerotic narrowing recurs, and the procedure needs to be repeated. A small proportion of these need further angioplasty at one year. Thereafter, the success rate is extremely high. With improved technique, the likelihood of the artery narrowing again will be markedly reduced. It is doubtful, however, that PTCA will be a complete substitute for bypass surgery. By present standards, I would hazard a guess that ultimately about 20 to 25% of surgical candidates will be suitable.

There have been conflicting reports on the benefits of angioplasty (PTCA) in women. Some have found a higher recurrence in narrowing rate at 6 and 12 months than in men and more complications occurring during the procedure itself. This has been explained on the basis of smaller arteries, more delicate vessel walls, and particularly in younger women, a more aggressive form of coronary disease. Others have not had the same experience and maintain that complications and recurrence are no more frequent than in men. As in CABG surgery, the long-term results are similar in both men and women.

In my experience, patients who undergo PTCA are likely to underestimate the chronic nature of their disease. They see the procedure as a quick fix and fail to recognize the necessity for rehabilitation. Whether a vigorously pursued rehabilitation program can keep the artery open remains a subject for further research. But many of the benefits obtained from rehabilitation by CABG patients are also applicable to those who have had the PTCA procedure.

Atherectomy Patients

Coronary atherectomy is a new procedure, not as yet carried out in all hospitals, but becoming more popular as familiarity with the technique spreads. A fine catheter with a slot on one side near the tip is inserted into the coronary artery. A blade that rotates at the rate of 1,000 rpm is contained in the catheter. The slot is brought in contact with the atherosclerotic plaque, and the blade shaves off the protruding atheroma (Figure 37). The catheter can be advanced down the obstructed segment of the coronary artery and then rotated so as to reduce the narrowing around the entire lumen of the coronary vessel. Since the catheters are not too flexible, they cannot enter tortuous areas of the coronary vessels, and their use is thus limited to lesions in the larger straight branches. The patient can usually leave the hospital the day after the procedure. Patients have the same needs for rehabilitation.

Heart Transplantation Patients

There have been exciting new developments in the area of heart transplantation. After some false and shaky starts in the 1970s (due largely to overly optimistic predictions and subsequent bad publicity), the 1980s saw the estab-

Figure 37: Atherectomy
A fine catheter containing a blade is inserted into the artery and the atheroma is shaved.

lishment of a firm foundation for future widespread success. The discovery of new medications to overcome the major problem of rejection has not only enabled the patient with a new heart to be out of hospital in a matter of weeks, but it has also improved the five-year survival rate to well above 70%. There are now more than 200 centers in the world performing over 3,000 heart transplants annually.

One of the leading centers in the world for heart transplant surgery is Harefield Hospital in London, England. The surgeon, Mr. Magdi Yacoub, is a firm advocate of postsurgical exercise rehabilitation, and in 1984, he and I set up a joint research project between Harefield and the Toronto Rehabilitation Centre. This program involved the exercise testing and training of English transplant patients by senior members of the Centre's staff. Every three months, they spent a week or so in Harefield working with the new patients and reassessing previous ones. In the intervals between these visits, communication was maintained by mailed exercise logs, in similar manner to the system adopted for patients on the TRC Outreach Program.

The results were excellent and were published in the official journal of the American Heart Association, *Circulation*, in 1988. A total of 36 patients trained for two years, the longest training period for heart transplant patients yet recorded. In the final months of training, they were averaging 13 miles (21 kilometers) of walking/jogging weekly; the eight most motivated subjects averaged in excess of 20 miles (32 kilometers). The average improvement in peak work load attained on exercise testing was 27% (54% for the high-mileage eight) and in peak oxygen intake 43% (64%). One of the patients entered the 26-mile (42-kilometer) Boston Marathon in 1985, 12 months after entering the training program and 15 months after undergoing the transplant procedure. He was the first transplant patient to do so.

Apart from these remarkable physiological gains, the training regime was associated with significant improvements in self-confidence, reduction in anxiety, and alleviation of depression; in short, vast enhancement in quality of life. There seems little doubt that heart transplant patients are ideal candidates for exercise rehabilitation.

Heart transplantation is carried out when the patient's life is threatened by severe heart failure. Since the commonest cause of failure is extensive coronary disease, fewer females are candidates for a heart replacement operation. In fact, the men outnumber the women by about six to one. The women also tend to be younger than the men. Although for some reason there is a tendency for women to have more episodes of rejection during the early post-surgical months, this does not affect their short- and long-term survival rate, which is the same as that for the men. Their response to an exercise rehabilitation program also corresponds closely to that for men.

Other Types of Patients

Patients recovering from *cardiac valve surgery*, whose surgery may have been a success but who are still disabled by years of presurgical restricted exercise and resultant deconditioning, are, in selected cases, suitable candidates for exercise rehabilitation. A point to be borne in mind is that some of these patients receive anti-clotting therapy and may not tolerate vigorous weight-bearing training activities. Also, some types of mechanical valves place some limitation, at least theoretically, on heart performance during maximal effort.

For many years it has been an established practice for patients who have suffered from *heart failure* or who have poorly functioning ventricles to avoid all exercise. However, in recent years the situation has been re-evaluated. Once out of the acute stage of failure and if there is no leg swelling or evidence of backup of fluid in the lungs, then a low-level, medically prescribed, carefully supervised exercise program has been shown to improve performance on the exercise test, increase oxygen intake, enhance functional capacity for all the activities of daily living, and markedly improve morale. The TRC program has a small number of these patients currently on a special pilot project. Experience is still limited, and research is continuing in a number of centers around the world. In the meantime, however, it would appear that a combination of the new heart failure drugs and a prudent exercise training regime can significantly improve these patients' outlook.

SAFETY OF EXERCISE REHABILITATION

Recognizing that patients with coronary heart disease, both those with or those without symptoms, are more likely to suffer a fatal heart attack or a cardiac arrest than their healthy counterparts, it is reassuring to know that the safety record of medically supervised cardiac exercise programs is excellent. Our experience at the Toronto Rehabilitation Centre now includes more than 3 million documented exercise sessions. During that time, there has been one non-fatal and one fatal exercise-related heart attack for every 610,562 and 508,802 sessions respectively, a low incidence for even a coronary-free healthy population.

We have adopted a number of routine precautionary measures at the TRC in order to minimize the risk of an accident. The supervising staff is not only efficient and observant, but works hard to create an informal and friendly atmosphere during exercise sessions so as to avoid feelings of tension or anxiety. The patients are also advised to adhere to the following exercise rules:

- always warm up and cool down;
- avoid extremes of heat and cold;
- train regularly without excessive peaks of activity;
- avoid intensive competition;
- adhere to the prescribed limits;
- reduce the exercise load when symptoms such as angina or frequent skipped beats occur, or during times when anxiety or tension is present; and
- report all symptoms, and particularly episodes of light-headedness or blackouts, no matter how brief.

WHO SHOULD NOT EXERCISE?

The vast majority of coronary heart disease patients, whether they have had a heart attack or suffer from angina, will benefit from a medically prescribed sensible exercise program. So also will the middle-aged individual who has any of the coronary risk factors (and that means most of us over the age of 40), or who has a family history of heart disease. There are, however, some people who should absolutely not exercise either for cardiac or non-cardiac reasons. Other people need to take extreme care. Exercise is possible for them, but it must be modified and adjusted to make it safe.

Cardiac Contraindications to Exercise

As I have said, these are few, and your physician should be your final guide.

1. A *recent heart attack*. Since the myocardial infarction scar takes about four to six weeks to become firm, vigorous activity prior to that time may cause a thinning of the scarred wall. If this occurs, the wall will become weak and bulge outwards every time the healthy muscle wall surrounding it contracts inwards. This bulge is known as an aneurysm. If the aneurysm is small, it is of little consequence. However, if the aneurysm is large, it can weaken the pumping power of the heart, a condition that may be associated with dangerous irregularities of heart beat. A large aneurysm can also prevent safe participation in a good exercise training program in the future. In most cases, a large aneurysm can be cured surgically by cutting out the thinned scarred area.

   This is not to say that normal activities of daily living, including comfortable walking, should not be permitted before the six-week period, but entry into a supervised training program should not take place until after a good exercise test.

2. There is no role for exercise in *acute heart failure*. In this condition, the heart is unable to pump the blood around the body efficiently; the symptoms are extreme breathlessness and swelling, or oedema, of the legs. Heart failure is not a common complication of coronary artery disease, but when it does occur, it is usually in association with a very severe heart attack resulting in extensive

damage to the heart muscle. Even then, healing of the infarct may result in complete recovery in pump efficiency, at which time exercise again becomes permissible. In recent years, patients who have suffered from attacks of heart failure and have been stabilized by some of the newer medications, are undertaking carefully monitored exercise rehabilitation programs with promising results. However, more research is needed in this area, and until we have accumulated additional information, these patients should not be encouraged to exercise on their own. Their place is in a specialized center under the guidance of skilled exercise specialists.

3. As we have seen, a *large aneurysm* of the heart wall is a bar to exercise. Aneurysms may also occur in the walls of the large blood vessels (for example, the aorta), and their presence here also precludes vigorous training. There are, of course, cases in which small aneurysmal bulges are present; here the question of whether or not to exercise becomes a matter of fine judgment. Again, such individuals should not attempt to regulate their own program, and skilled supervision by a physician is essential.

4. Patients who develop *rapidly progressing anginal pain* should not exercise. Any change for the worse in the *pattern* and *incidence* of exertional pain may well be the warning of another heart attack. A typical example might be a patient who finds that angina is induced at a much lower level of exertion than usual. Or, alternatively, a patient who generally suffers from exertional angina only, but then finds that he or she is being awakened during the night with chest pain. To exercise under these circumstances may well be to invite disaster.

5. The heart muscle can sometimes be involved in *generalized infections*, giving rise to a condition known as myocarditis, or inflammation of the myocardium (the medical ending "itis" means "inflammation of"). This infection can occur

in acute rheumatic fever, or in viral infections such as infectious mononucleosis (glandular fever) or even influenza. Since exercise is never advised during acute infections, it is obviously even more dangerous when the infection involves the heart. While your physician will be the one to diagnose myocarditis and will certainly ensure that your physical activity is limited until the condition has cleared, it should be stressed that mild subclinical myocarditis may be common in association with a number of viral-type infections. For this reason, I insist that all individuals on an exercise program stop training whenever they develop any influenza-like illness, particularly one that is accompanied by muscle pain, tenderness, and a rapid heart rate. Exercise should never be performed in the presence of a fever, and to be on the safe side, the temperature should have returned to normal for a full seven days before working out again.

6. *Markedly irregular heart action* that is aggravated by exertion is a deterrent to training, especially if the electrocardiogram shows that these ectopic beats are emanating from more than one area in the heart. These "multi-focal" ectopics, which are aggravated by strenuous exertion, can on occasion lead to fatal ventricular fibrillation, and exercise should not be undertaken until the condition has been controlled by suitable medication. Compensation can be made for lesser degrees of rhythm irregularity by modifying the training regimen.

It should be stressed that there can also be benign irregularities in the heartbeat. These are often present from youth. The distinction can only be made accurately if they are seen on an electrocardiogram, but a rough rule of thumb to their identification is that these irregularities are often present at rest but disappear as the heart rate increases with exercise.

7. In certain types of *valvular heart disease*, especially those that lead to severe narrowing in the region of the aortic valve, exercise training may not be advisable. Coronary heart disease does not affect the valves in this manner; rheumatic fever in childhood is the usual offender. Occasionally, both valvular disease and coronary artery disease can co-exist, in which case one has to be guided by the severity of the valvular difficulty.

8. Patients suffering from recent cases of *blood clots* occurring either in the lungs (pulmonary embolism), or in the peripheral arteries or veins (thrombophlebitis), should not be exercising. Physical activity may bring about further clots, or extension of the existing ones.

9. *Repeated bouts of heart failure* may, in the long run, give rise to a dilated enlarged heart. This will show up on the X-ray and also on an echocardiogram. Where the enlargement is pronounced, there will be no benefit from training. The stretched heart muscle has no reserve left and so is incapable of benefiting from even measured small doses of exercise stress.

10. Exercise therapy is of little value in the condition of *complete heart block*. Here, the electrical conduction system between the upper and lower chambers of the heart is non-functioning, with the result that the atria and the ventricles beat independently. Furthermore, an increase in heart rate does not occur when the subject exercises. In such a condition, a pacemaker, or artificial rhythm conductor, is inserted. This brings the heart rate up to a set level and may also, depending on the type and design, permit it to accelerate in response to exercise. Those individuals who have been fitted with an appropriate pacemaker can benefit from an exercise program.

11. Most patients with high blood pressure do well on an exercise program. However, if the *hypertension* is very

marked, *in excess of 200/100 mm Hg*, and cannot be controlled by medication, then vigorous exercise is harmful because it drives the pressure up higher and may cause a stroke.

12. Certain forms of *congenital heart disease*, especially those that are associated with a bluish discoloration of the face, feet, and hands (cyanosis), are contraindicators to exercise.

Non-Cardiac Contraindications to Exercise

1. If you suffer from *severe uncontrolled diabetes*, you should avoid undue physical exertion until your condition is stabilized.

2. Some individuals suffering from *epilepsy* may find that exercise, by bringing the body to a state of "arousal," may increase the frequency of seizures. In such cases, the problem may be solved by altering the dosage or type of anti-seizure medication, or by modifying the intensity or duration of the training session. Often a satisfactory modification can be achieved by a process of trial and error.

3. Sustained exercise makes increased demands on the lungs, kidneys, and liver, and in *diseases* where the functions of these organs are severely compromised, exercise is obviously contraindicated.

4. The acute stages of various types of *arthritis*, such as rheumatoid arthritis or gout, are treated by appropriate medication and rest. During these acute phases, exercise will do more harm than good. However, during the quiescent phase, suitably modified exercise programs will be beneficial.

   The more crippling type of osteoarthritis may be aggravated by weight-bearing activities such as running or jogging; in these situations cycling or swimming may be more appropriate. In passing, however, I should note that long-distance runners have been shown to have a lower incidence of osteoarthritis in their hip joints than the population at large; this is due to the fact that movement keeps the protective cartilaginous lining of the joint surfaces healthy and well nourished. Our legs were meant for walking — not sitting.

5. *Chronic low back trouble* can be exacerbated by jogging or by certain types of calisthenics. However, factors that are even more aggravating are obesity, running on an uneven surface, wearing unsuitable running shoes, or performing activities that involve twisting movements of the spine: the golf drive, the tennis serve, squash, or badminton. If a careful watch is kept for flare-ups, and activity is slowed with the advent of suspicious symptoms, back strength should develop to the stage where a full program of walking/jogging can be sustained without problems.

6. There are a number of other conditions in which exercise may be ill-advised. These include various rare neurological, muscular, and glandular diseases. In any event, the physician must be the final judge in these matters, and his or her advice and permission are essential for any patient with coronary heart disease who wishes to embark upon the training system outlined in this book.

9. The Benefits of Exercise Rehabilitation

We have already dealt with exercise training as a way of reducing or eliminating many of the risk factors for coronary disease. We have also seen that the training reduces resting and exercise heart rates, increases the amount of blood the heart can eject with each beat, reduces resting and exercising blood pressure, enhances the efficiency with which the muscles can extract oxygen, and increases maximal oxygen intake. We will now look at the extent to which these changes apply to the cardiac rehabilitation patient.

Psychological

A person who survives a heart attack frequently suffers from mental depression. Even after physical recovery is apparently complete, this problem may continue. Psychological evaluation of patients referred to the TRC program has consistently shown that between one-third and one-half can have quite profound depression. Happily, however, we have found a considerable improvement after just one year of training. A four-year follow-up of 44 of our most severely depressed subjects showed a significant 13% reduction in their depression score, which related directly to compliance with our exercise program.

In another study, 317 male post-heart attack patients who completed one year of training had less tension and hostility as well as more confidence and increased feelings of vigor. More recently, we have been working with heart transplant patients, and here the effects of training have been quite dramatic. A two-year follow-up of 30 transplant patients entered into the program showed that, while initially depressed and anxious, their training was accompanied by a significant lessening of depression, a decrease in anxiety and fatigue, and an increase in vigor.

Heart Performance

Since the heart is a major link in the oxygen transport chain, it is not surprising that patients admitted to the program after a heart attack frequently have a low maximal oxygen intake on the initial exercise test. Over the course of the program, they show an average increase in VO_2max of 25%. A higher VO_2max means more than just an improved performance in a laboratory test; it means an increased capacity to lead a full active life.

RELIEF OF ANGINA

The symptom of angina (or the development of ST segment depression on the electrocardiogram, referred to as *silent angina*) is the result of an imbalance between supply and demand; in other words, it occurs when the heart is working so hard that it outstrips the ability of its coronary arteries to supply it with an adequate flow of oxygenated blood. In the case of someone with coronary arteries narrowed because of atherosclerosis, it may not take too much work on the part of the heart for the demand to exceed the supply.

If we want to cure angina, or reduce ST segment depression, we can, at least theoretically, approach the problem in two ways. We can either *reduce the demand* imposed by the heart on the narrowed coronaries, or we can *increase the blood supply* to the heart through the coronaries. Immediate short-term relief of angina can be provided by the use of nitroglycerine, which *temporarily* dilates the coronary arteries, thereby increasing the supply, while at the same time dilating the arteries and veins throughout the body, dropping the pressure against which the heart has to work, and thus reducing the demand. The beta-blockers, which drop heart rate and blood pressure at all levels of effort, also prevent angina, but only by decreasing the heart's demand for blood.

One of the most consistently reported benefits of exercise training in patients is the eventual relief of exertional angina and the reduction of ST segment depression as seen on the exercise electrocardiogram. It sounds paradoxical that exercise training can cure a symptom that is itself brought on by exercise. Does training work by reducing demand, increasing supply, or both?

Reduction in Demand

Exertional angina generally occurs at a particular Rate Pressure Product (heart rate × systolic blood pressure). This RPP is referred to as the patient's anginal threshold. Because training reduces the heart rate and blood pressure, eventually the patient can reproduce that same level of work without reaching the RPP anginal threshold. The heart's demand for blood has been reduced.

A typical example is the patient who gets anginal pain when walking a mile (1.6 kilometers) in, say, 20 minutes. At that pace, the heart rate increases to perhaps 110 beats per minute, and the systolic blood pressure to 130 mm Hg, giving an RPP of 14,300 (110 × 130). Let us say that after training for two months, the 20-minute walk can now be accomplished at a heart rate of 102 beats per minute and a systolic blood pressure of 126 mm Hg. The RPP is now 12,852, well below the anginal threshold (Figure 38). Ultimately, the patient is able to carry out all the normal activities of daily life, including vigorous activities, without ever reaching the anginal threshold.

Increase in Supply

There is another mechanism by which training can reduce the symptom of angina. You will recall that blood flows through the coronary arteries during the period of diastole, the relaxation phase between heartbeats. A trained slow-beating heart has longer periods of diastole, thus allowing more time for coronary blood flow to occur. This additional circulation time is often sufficient to compensate for the reduction in flow caused by atherosclerotic narrowing. In a sense, this is a way of increasing supply.

From time to time, coronary patients become so fit that when we exercise-test them, they achieve a heart rate and blood pressure (Rate Pressure Product) higher than their previous anginal threshold and yet do not develop angina or ST segment changes (Figure 38). This indicates that, despite the increase in demand, the supply remains adequate. Therefore, the ability of the coronary circulation to provide the heart with blood must have improved. There are two ways this could happen. Either there has been growth of new coronary artery branches that detour the blood flow around the narrowed segment (like a natural bypass), or the narrowing itself has opened up as a result of shrinkage in the size of the atheromatous deposit. The first process is referred to as *collateralization*, and the second as *regression*.

Coronary collaterals are tiny blood vessels, no thicker than a fine hair, which vary in length from a few millimeters to about 3 centimeters. Under normal circumstances, they carry little or no blood. However, if the coronaries start to become narrowed as a result of atherosclerosis, then they respond to this by gradually growing in size and number

Figure 38: How Exercise Training Relieves Angina
This patient reaches the Rate Pressure Product (heart rate x blood pressure), which produces angina at a walking pace of three miles per hour (A). After three months of training, the resting and exercising RPP drops, and the anginal threshold is not reached until a pace of three-and-a-half miles per hour is attained (B). After six months, four miles per hour is attained before the onset of angina (C). Here, angina is being relieved by a reduction in cardiac work (RPP) at a given level of effort, i.e., a reduction in *demand*. Sometimes a patient becomes so fit that he can exercise to an RPP which is *greater* than the anginal threshold, yet experience no symptoms (D), circumstantial evidence that there has been an increase in *supply*, i.e., coronary blood flow has improved.

so as to compensate for any reduction in coronary blood flow. The greater the growth in collaterals (collateralization), the less likely is the coronary narrowing to cause angina, or to lead to a heart attack if the narrowing closes off altogether. Animal studies have shown that regular exercise training is a powerful stimulus to collateralization. As the animal becomes fitter, the collaterals increase in size and number (by the same token, when it stops training, the collateral vessels gradually shrink). Even when the animal is entered into an exercise training program *after* an experimentally induced heart attack, extensive collateralization is still seen, and this has been shown to improve survival from subsequent attacks.

The evidence for training-induced collateralization in humans has been less easy to obtain, mainly because the size and location of the collateral vessels make them difficult to see on a coronary angiogram. More recently, the technique of thallium exercise testing has shown evidence of collateral growth in coronary patients entered into an exercise rehabilitation program. As these techniques improve and coronary angiography becomes more sophisticated, we hope we will see more results of this type.

Regression, or reversal of coronary atherosclerosis by shrinking the atheromatous deposit, was first demonstrated in rabbit studies in which high-fat diet-induced atheromas gradually went away when a normal diet was reintroduced. The proof that regression could occur in human coronaries had to wait until the 1980s, when refinements in the technique of measuring the size of a deposit by coronary angiography were introduced. Presently, reports of regression occurring in coronary patients are few, but undoubtedly more will follow. In 1987 Dr. David Blankenhorn and his colleagues from the University of Southern California demonstrated regression of coronary atherosclerosis in a small group of patients who were following a low-fat diet and taking a combination of the bile resin, colestipol, and niacin.

Three years later Dr. Greg Brown and co-workers from the University of Washington reported similar results, the medication on this occasion being lovastatin. Dr. Dean Ornish and his group from the University of California described regression in the group of patients who followed a one-year rehabilitation-type program that included a vegetarian diet, daily exercise, and stress reduction techniques. In 1992, Dr. Gerhard Schuler and colleagues from the University Hospital in Heidelberg, Germany, reported significant regression of coronary atherosclerotic plaques in seven of eighteen patients who for one year followed the American Heart Association Step II diet, and carried out an exercise program that consisted of a minimum of 30 minutes of stationary cycling at home every day, and attendance at least twice a week at a 60-minute group workout. Neither the Ornish nor the Schuler study used cholesterol-lowering drugs. Although the combined number of patients in all of these trials is small, the results have been highly encouraging and similar larger studies are now under way around the world.

Retarding the Progression of Coronary Atherosclerosis
In coronary-prone populations, atherosclerotic deposits begin to appear at about age 20 years. Since 60% of the coronary blood vessels have to be involved in the disease process before circulation to the heart muscle is compromised and angina or a heart attack occurs, the rate at which the deposits increase in size is of paramount importance. For instance, starting at age 20, a 1% per annum increase would only begin to cause a problem at age 80 years, hardly a serious threat. On the other hand, a 3% per annum increase will lead to symptoms at age 40. Merely reducing the annual progression of the disease by 2%, which should be obtained by attacking the major risk factors, can make the difference between a long life and premature death.

The same applies to the patient who has already suffered a heart attack. If the disease can be arrested, or the rate of progression slowed, then the likelihood of future events is considerably reduced, or even eliminated.

SECONDARY PREVENTION

So far we have seen that an exercise program can greatly enhance the heart attack survivor's quality of life, improve functional capacity, counteract the risk factors for coronary heart disease, improve symptoms, and permit early return to work. For these reasons alone, exercise rehabilitation is strongly advocated by such bodies as the World Health Organization and, indeed, all the national and international heart foundations and associations.

In the final analysis, however, can we say that exercise training per se prevents a recurrent heart attack? From the outset, it has been the experience of all programs that recurrence rates are reduced. In a group of 2,500 post-coronary patients who had attended the TRC program, a 10-year follow-up revealed an annual fatal recurrence rate of 1.9%. This compared very favorably with the annual rate of 3% to 4% reported for sedentary patients who had not been referred for exercise rehabilitation. However, we wanted to investigate the possibility that our results might have been biased by the fact that the physicians had chosen to refer to the program only those patients most likely to benefit and had excluded those who were the most ill. In order to do this, we matched patients according to their smoking habits, blood cholesterol levels, and presence or absence of angina, hypertension, and diabetes. We then compared those who continued to exercise regularly with those who stopped exercising for non-medical reasons such as boredom, being too busy, and general lack of motivation. Analysis of the data revealed that the death rate from recurrent heart attack was 60% lower in the exercisers over the ten-year period.

A number of prospective randomized exercise trials have been carried out during the 1970s and the 1980s in order to address the question of secondary prevention. All have shown a reduction in the incidence of recurrent fatal heart attack in the exercisers, but the results have not always reached statistically significant levels. The reason for this has been the inadequate number of subjects and the short period of follow-up, both the results of inadequate funding.

Given the problems of inadequate numbers and short follow-up that have typified the randomized exercise trials, the most reasonable approach has been to use meta-analysis. This was first carried out by Dr. Graham May and his colleagues, who pooled the data from a number of randomized trials and found a statistically significant 19% reduction in total mortality as a result of exercise training. Dr. Neil Oldridge and his co-workers from Ontario combined the results of ten randomized clinical trials and found a 25% reduction in recurrent fatal heart attacks in the exercising group.

The most recent overview and analysis of 22 randomized trials has come from Dr. Gerald O'Connor and his colleagues, who also found that exercise programs reduced the risk of fatal recurrence by 20% and the risk of sudden death by as much as 37%.

I think it is fair to say that we now have evidence that a carefully prescribed and supervised postcoronary exercise training program plays a major role in reducing fatal recurrence rates and sudden cardiac death. Since the rehabilitation program also includes advice on diet, smoking, diabetes, and appropriate medications, the combined effect of all these strategies is bound to significantly reduce deaths from recurrent heart attacks.

10. Your Exercise Prescription

As a result of more than 25 years' experience training thousands of coronary heart disease patients at the Toronto Rehabilitation Centre, we have developed a plan that, followed carefully and sensibly, will provide a safe and effective method of developing endurance fitness. However, let me start with a word of warning. Circumstances and individuals vary. Mindless adherence to this or any other training system could have unpleasant consequences, especially for those with coronary heart disease. While training usually leads to improved health and heart function, coronary disease can occasionally become unstable. The warning signs and symptoms of such deterioration are described on pages 242-243. If they become apparent, the exercise prescription should be reduced immediately. Similarly, if you have difficulty completing the prescribed workout, you should modify the requirements to suit your own tolerance. If in doubt, talk to your physician. *Prudence takes precedence over enthusiasm when you are training a damaged heart!*

With these precautions in mind, let's take a closer look at the training tables reproduced in the appendices. They consist of three phases.

Phase 1

The point at which you start your training depends on your fitness level, as determined by your maximum oxygen intake and your age. If your initial maximal oxygen intake (VO_2max) is less than 16 mL/kg per minute (and we will see later how to measure this), you should carry out a preliminary phase that lasts for eight weeks. In addition, those who are overweight, have been sedentary for many years, or suffer from musculoskeletal problems such as low back pain or mild osteoarthritis in their knees or hips should also adhere to the eight-week breaking-in period — even though their initial fitness may be higher than the specified level.

If your VO_2max is higher than 16 mL, your initial goal should be a 3-mile (5-kilometer) walk. The speed of the walk will be determined by your level of fitness. The 3 miles (5 kilometers) should be approached in stages: for two weeks, walk 1 mile (1.6 kilometers); for the next two weeks, walk 2 miles (3 kilometers); and finally, walk the 3 miles (5 kilometers), all at the prescribed speed. After that, you will progress to the next level by walking the 3-mile (5-kilometer) distance at a faster pace.

Try to walk five times a week, with two days' rest. It's immaterial whether these rest days are taken together, or split. The choice is a matter of personal convenience.

I should point out that the maximal oxygen intake levels used in Phase 1 were derived from an exercise test carried out at the Centre on patients suffering from coronary artery disease.

Phase 2

In this phase, the intensity of the workout is slowly increased to a desired pace. If you are under the age of 45 and free from coronary heart disease or any of its manifestations, the pace is 10 minutes per mile (6 minutes per kilometer);

if over 45, or suffering from coronary heart disease or any of its manifestations, then the pace is 12 minutes per mile (7.5 minutes per kilometer). When you achieve your desired pace, the distance is lengthened to 4 miles (6.5 kilometers), at the same speed. This phase is crucial and may take many months to complete; if you suffer from coronary heart disease, you should be particularly alert for such adverse symptoms as chest pain, extreme breathlessness, irregular heart action, or lightheadedness during the workout. If the condition of your heart is unstable, the instability is more likely to reveal itself at the quicker pace.

For most of us, walking faster than 15 minutes per mile (9.5 minutes per kilometer) or 4 miles (6.5 kilometers) per hour is a waste of energy and excessively strenuous. To avoid this strain, short jogging segments are added to the training when the prescription calls for a 14.5 minutes-per-mile (9-minutes-per-kilometer) pace. This is done gradually through each of five stages until one attains a 12 minutes-per-mile (7.5-minutes-per-kilometer) pace, at which time the entire distance of 3 miles (5 kilometers) is jogged (see Appendix B).

The jogging technique is described in detail later. At this stage it is sufficient to say that it should be relaxed, flat-footed and with short strides; the speed should be little above that of a walk. Actually, I think the term "plodding" is more descriptive than jogging.

Phase 3
In Phase 3, you progress to jogging 6 miles (10 kilometers) in 60 or 72 minutes, depending on your age and whether you are suffering from coronary heart disease. It takes about 12 months to reach this goal. Anyone who has managed to progress through the first two phases and is free from symptoms and signs should be able to finish Phase 3, but it should be undertaken only by those who really enjoy jogging. Jogging for an hour a day, five times a week is

time-consuming and is not for everyone, but it pays off in a high level of cardiorespiratory fitness. From the ranks of the "one-hour joggers" have come many postcoronary marathoners. Nonetheless, this phase is strictly optional.

HOW TO USE THE TABLES

Determining Your Starting Level

How fit are you? The only way to answer this accurately is to take a formal exercise test, which will measure your aerobic power, or maximal oxygen intake. The test will also indicate any electrocardiographic abnormalities that develop during training sessions. Such a test is mandatory for all patients entering my exercise rehabilitation program. If you are a would-be exerciser and have a heart problem, ask your physician to arrange an exercise test. If he or she doesn't do this procedure, ask to be referred to a physician who does.

If you have had a heart attack, or suffer from angina pectoris or palpitations and there are no facilities for exercise testing in your area, then to ensure your safety, start at the very beginning of the training tables, that is, at Level 1 of the Preliminary Phase. Again, you should pursue this course *only if you have had prior clearance from your physician.*

If you are healthy and would like to determine your aerobic fitness level, your first step should be to complete the Physical Activity Readiness Questionnaire (see Appendix F). This was designed for use before taking the Canadian Standardized Test of Fitness, a similar submaximal bench test to the one about to be described. If you pass this questionnaire — that is, if you answer no to all the questions — then proceed as follows.

Submaximal Step Test

The following submaximal step test is one devised by Professor Roy Shephard, and I am indebted to him for its use here. The procedure requires you to step up and down two steps of 9 inches (23 centimeters) each, to a count of six. Keep your feet flat and stand up straight. Start with the feet together on the ground, then left foot on the first step — count one; right foot on the second step — count two; left foot joins right foot — count three; right foot on the first step — count four; left foot on the ground — count five; right foot joins left foot — count six. The lead leg can be alternated every other minute to reduce fatigue.

The rate of stepping is important since it affects the energy cost of the test. Our aim is an effort intensity about 75% of maximum. This will, of course, vary with age and body weight, and therefore Appendix G gives the appropriate tempo in terms of steps per minute, as well as the energy cost of this effort in milliliters of oxygen per kilogram per minute. The accompanying table also shows the 75% age-related anticipated heart rate after three minutes of stepping; this rate is based on the normal sedentary population and is accurate to within plus or minus ten beats per minute.

Once you have worked out the correct stepping rate for your age and weight, practice with a stopwatch until you get the tempo, then step up and down for three minutes. Your aim is to attain your approximate target heart rate within that time. Immediately on stopping, take a ten-second pulse count (see pages 243-245 for instructions). With this figure, using the appropriate age-related nomogram (Appendix A) you can calculate your maximal oxygen intake.

A line joining your energy cost of stepping and your exercise heart rate will intersect the center line at your estimated maximal oxygen intake, expressed in milliliters of oxygen. Dividing this by your weight in kilograms (1 kilogram = 2.2 pounds) will give you your maximal oxygen intake expressed in milliliters of oxygen per kilogram per minute. Apply this figure to Phase I of the training tables, and you have your starting level of training.

Let us say you are a 45-year-old male who weighs 160 pounds (72 kilograms). Appendix G tells you to carry out the step test at the rate of 102 steps per minute to utilize 1,885 milliliters of oxygen per minute, which, for the average sedentary individual of that age and weight, would be equivalent to three-quarters of all-out effort. As a further check, the resultant pulse rate for that degree of effort (75% of maximum) is obtained from the accompanying table, i.e., 140 beats per minute plus or minus 10 beats.

You now carry out the test at the required rate of stepping for three minutes. At the end of this time you take your ten-second pulse count. Let us say it comes to 25 beats in 10 seconds, or 150 beats per minute. Then, from nomogram E you read off a predicted maximal oxygen intake of 2,200 milliliters per minute (a line joining 1,885 on the right column and 150 on the left column intersects the center sloping line at 2,200). You divide your predicted maximal oxygen intake of 2,200 by your weight in kilograms (72) and you obtain a VO_2max corrected for weight of 30.3 mL/kg per minute. Applying this to the training tables would mean that you start at Level 7 of Phase 1, or 3 miles (5 kilometers) in 45 minutes.

This might sound complicated but it is easier to do than to describe. However, if you find it a chore even to contemplate, then skip it and start at the Preliminary Phase, Level 1.

Some Warnings

If you develop chest pain or discomfort, extreme breathlessness, lightheadedness, or other adverse symptoms before the three minutes are up, stop immediately and note your pulse rate. It will represent your maximal heart rate for training purposes. For safety's sake, obtain your doctor's permission before you start the exercise program. If he or she agrees that exercise can help you, then start at the preliminary conditioning stage of the tables, and be sure that your pulse rate during the workout remains at least ten beats per minute below the symptom-producing level.

If after two minutes or so of stepping, you feel that you cannot continue because your legs are too tired, stop. You are even less fit than the average sedentary person of your age and weight. If you take your pulse rate at the time that you have to stop, you will find that it is already well above target rate. Don't despair, try again the following day, but this time choose the next lowest tempo listed in the table, e.g., 96 instead of 102 steps per minute.

Two very important points! Your stepping rate must be as accurately timed as possible. The best way to do this is to use a simple metronome, the sort that piano teachers use. Secondly, pulse rate should be obtained immediately on stopping. Ideally it should be taken during the last minute of the test, but this is very difficult to do. Instead, as you stop, take a ten-second pulse count, and then multiply the result by six to give a full minute's count. Remember, heart rate begins to drop rapidly with the cessation of exercise, and if you delay as little as even 30 seconds in finding and counting your pulse, the result will not truly represent your heart rate in the final minutes of the test.

Finally, at the risk of being unduly repetitive, let me once again warn you against attempting this or any other self-administered test without the permission of your physician — especially if you have any symptoms of coronary artery disease. Paradoxically, those most curious to know their fitness level are the overweight, sedentary, obviously unfit members of the population — precisely those in whom atherosclerosis is likely to be present. Beware that curiosity doesn't kill the fat cat.

Taking Your Pulse Count

It is essential that you take your pulse accurately. As the beating heart ejects its blood into the aorta, the impulse is transmitted down the aorta's walls to all of its branches, where it is felt as a pulse. Thus, the pulse rate coincides with the heart rate. Physicians traditionally measure heart rate by timing the pulse of the radial artery, which is felt in the front of the wrist just below the base of the thumb. At this point the radial artery lies just beneath the skin and is easily felt because it can be steadied against the underlying wrist bones. Exercise physiologists tend to use the carotid pulse, the large artery in the front of the neck, which can be felt on either side of the Adam's apple; this vessel pumps very vigorously during exercise, and for that reason is easier to obtain.

Use whichever you find the easiest. If you use the carotid, however, be careful not to press too hard, otherwise you will press on a structure known as the carotid sinus, which will slow the heart rate momentarily. The advantage of taking the carotid pulse is that it allows you to operate a stopwatch in the other hand and so get an accurate count. If you are having difficulty in feeling the carotid pulse, you may be throwing your head back, a movement that causes the carotid arteries to move away from the front of the neck. If you want to feel the carotid pulse easily, then hold your head in the normal position, or even tilt it slightly forward.

Since you are counting for only ten seconds and multiplying by six, accuracy is essential. For uniformity's sake, we tell our patients to start counting "zero, one, two, three," etc., the zero marking the commencement of the ten-second count.

Why count for only ten seconds? Ideally, we want to know what the heart rate is *during* the exercise session. As soon as you start to work out, your resting heart rate climbs, and within two or three minutes reaches a plateau that remains steady for as long as you exercise — provided, of course, that you maintain the same pace. It is impractical to take the pulse rate while jogging, or even walking, but for 10 or 15 seconds after you stop your heart rate will remain at the plateau. Pulse rates, then, taken within ten seconds of stopping jogging or brisk walking, are a fairly accurate measure of the heart rate during the workout. Thereafter, the rate drops off rapidly. If you wait for even as short a time as 20 seconds to take your count, it will no longer be representative of the rate during exercise.

When to Move From One Phase to the Next
The tables are designed to train you at an intensity of approximately 50% to 70% of your maximal oxygen intake or, expressed another way, 60% to 80% of your maximal heart rate. As you become fitter, however, both your resting and your exercising pulse rates will become slower. Eventually, the intensity and duration of the prescribed workout will no longer obtain the required training pulse rate. When this stage is reached, progression to a higher level is indicated. Use nomogram A to determine this point. To use this nomogram, you need to know your resting and exercise pulse rates. Your maximal heart rate has already been estimated from age-related tables. Your resting pulse rate is taken immediately on awakening in the morning and before you get out of bed or after sitting relaxed in an armchair for five minutes or so.

When the prescribed walk/jog consistently fails to achieve the progressing pulse rate for a period of two weeks, then the time has come to move up to the next level of the table. Say, for instance, that a 40-year-old woman who started at Level 5, Phase 1 (3 miles or 4.8 kilometers in 48 minutes) had a resting pulse rate of 72 beats per minute. To use nomogram A, she would take a piece of dark thread and place one end at 72 on the resting heart rate column (values less than 72 can, for the purposes of prediction, be ignored). She would then stretch the thread to the 40 on the age column. The point where the thread crosses the center line is her progressing heart rate: 130 beats per minute. Thus, when her pulse count in the ten seconds following her three-mile (4.8-kilometer) walk is at or below this level of 130 consistently for a period of two weeks (an average of ten successive workouts), she would be ready to progress to Level 6 (3 miles or 4.8 kilometers in 45 minutes). The use of the nomogram, therefore, enables safe and effective progression without constant retesting. It gives an element of objectivity to the training regime; instead of stepping up your program because you feel fit and well, you can apply a physiological measure to validate your enthusiasm.

To get maximal value from the nomogram, you must use it correctly. Not only must the exercise pulse rate be at or below the progressing heart rate *consistently* for ten or more exercise sessions but progression to a higher level of effort should not be attempted if you are experiencing any of the signs of overtraining such as excessive tiredness, palpitations (premature ventricular beats), or muscle aches and pains. Your pulse rate must be charted at the end of each exercise session in order to keep an accurate record.

Of course, the nomogram contains two other variables, age and resting pulse rate. The majority of people reach the end of Phase 2 within a two-year period; therefore, once you have started on the program, it should not be necessary to change your age level on the left-hand column. As for resting pulse rate, this also drops with training, but the change is more variable than with exercise pulse rate. For patients on a supervised program, a new resting pulse rate can be established at the time of each laboratory exercise test; failing this, it is a good idea to check your resting pulse rate every three to six months and adjust the right-hand column accordingly.

If You Have Angina Pectoris
So far, we have been discussing the use of the nomogram to check the progress of the individual who does not suffer from symptoms such as angina pectoris. What of the patient who suffers from symptoms, especially when exercising? For this individual, there is a special nomogram. Into this

category also fall those patients whose formal exercise test revealed the presence of such ECG abnormalities as ST segment depression, exercise-induced frequent extrasystoles (see page 251), or some other complication (see Appendix A).

A hospital-type program with regular exercise testing can determine the exact level of exertion at which cardiac problems develop. Such repeated testing may be impractical, however, in a home program. A more individualized approach has therefore been developed that takes into account the pulse rate at which untoward symptoms or signs develop. Nomogram B permits the choice of a suitable starting level of exercise for the patient with symptoms and assures his or her subsequent safe progress through the various stages of the tables.

To use this nomogram, note must be made of the pulse rate at which the symptoms developed during an exercise test, either carried out in the doctor's office or at home. This is the maximum heart rate, symptom limited, or maxHR^{SL}. Using this figure, together with the resting pulse rate (obtained as previously), the training pulse rate can be read from nomogram B.

A word of warning: If the difference between your resting pulse rate and your maxHR^{SL} is 40 beats per minute or less, you should exercise only under the strict supervision of a physician. As you can see from the nomogram, the spread between training and progressing heart rates would be small in your case, requiring careful, accurate professional monitoring.

If this proviso does not apply to you, a trial one-mile (1.6-kilometer) walk is then taken, at a pace that is considered brisk, but not so fast as to bring on chest pain, skipped beats, or undue breathlessness. The pulse rate is taken in the ten seconds immediately following the walk and is compared with the desired training pulse rate. Depending on the result, the pace is adjusted to the nearest appropriate level in Phase 1. Always err on the side of safety: keep the intensity of exercise below the level at which symptoms develop. It may take one or two sessions to select the desired pace, but with patience and care, it is surprising how accurate one can be.

The following example will illustrate the method. Assume you have a resting heart rate of 72 beats per minute. While being tested, you develop evidence of myocardial ischaemia, say chest pain, at a heart rate of 124 beats per minute. This means you have a maxHR^{SL} of 124. From the nomogram, you determine that your training heart rate^{SL} is 110 beats per minute. You now go for a trial 1-mile (1.6-kilometer) walk, choosing a level course, and keeping the pace slow enough to avoid chest pain or undue breathlessness. At the end of the measured mile (1.6 kilometers), which took you 20 minutes to cover, your immediate postexercise pulse rate is 108 beats per minute. This, then, is your starting level (Level 1, Phase 1 for the under 45-year-old). Over the next six weeks, you will progress to 2 miles (3.2 kilometers) and then to 3 miles (4.8 kilometers), keeping the same pace of 20 minutes per mile (12.5 minutes per kilometer). Using the same nomogram, you can also tell what your progressing pulse rate should be (in this example, 100 beats per minute). After each workout, you chart your pulse rate, and when this consistently fails to achieve 100 beats per minute for ten consecutive sessions, and provided you have none of the adverse symptoms mentioned above, then you progress to Level 2, Phase 1.

I feel that complicated cases should be exercise tested every three months or so in order to have an objective measurement of improvement. When they can complete a test without adverse signs or symptoms, then they can proceed in accordance with nomogram A. Complicated cases require much closer physician supervision than uncomplicated ones, and the individuals ideally should be enrolled in a formal postcoronary exercise rehabilitation class where they can be watched during supervised exercise sessions and monitored frequently during the workouts.

In the early stages, the individual with symptoms during exercise will progress at a slower rate than his or her symptomless colleagues. This is to be expected and should not be allowed to cause discouragement or depression. Above all, any temptation to progress faster than the tables indicate should be vigorously resisted. You cannot bully a damaged heart. This is one game where breaking the rules may mean more than the loss of a few yards or a few points; it may mean "game over" for the only player involved — yourself! So, have patience, and remember that if it took 20 years to get out of shape, you can't really expect to regain your fitness in a few months.

If You are Taking Medication

Individuals who are taking a beta-blocker may have resting heart rates in the low fifties, with an accompanying reduction in heart rate at all levels of exertion, up to and including maximum. Therefore, attempts to achieve heart rates, either during exercise testing or workouts, based on age-related tables may be disastrous. For this reason, I place all patients taking a beta-blocker in the complicated category and use nomogram B for establishing both training heart rate and progressing heart rate. We have found this procedure to work well and have demonstrated repeatedly that patients who are taking beta-blockers can obtain a significant training effect. Of course, as they develop a training bradycardia (slow heart rate), their resting and working heart rates drop, and this reduction may be increased by the effect of the medication. Rather than having the resting heart rate become too slow, we customarily wait until it reaches the forties and then request the patient's cardiologist to consider reducing the beta-blocker dosage. This usually results in a return of the resting rate to the mid or high fifties. As training continues, the rate eventually returns to the forties again, and once more the dosage may be reduced. Eventually the medication may be stopped altogether or may be continued in small doses for its secondary preventive effect.

Ideally, patients on a beta-blocker should try to exercise at approximately the same time each day. This will ensure that the blood levels of the medication are approximately the same during each workout, and therefore pulse rates will be stable.

Since beta-blockers relieve angina by reducing the Rate Pressure Product for a given level of effort, and since exercise training seems to produce the same result by way of the same mechanism, I am sometimes asked, "Why exercise? Why not just use the drug to get fit?" Apart from the fact that exercise training has fewer contraindications and side effects, the beta-blocker lowers *maximal* heart rate and blood pressure and so, unlike exercise training, may limit physical performance. Of course, where angina is preventing everyday submaximal levels of activity, relief by a beta-blocker can for all practical purposes enhance physical capacity.

Calcium channel blockers do not interfere with the training effect, and they are mentioned here primarily because of their effect on pulse rate. Adalat and Cardene, the most commonly used for hypertension, will frequently increase pulse rate, and for this reason may often be given in conjunction with a beta-blocker. Cardizem slows pulse rate, although not as dramatically as the beta-blockers. Finally, Isoptin either has no effect or reduces pulse rate.

Digitalis is a drug that often reduces the resting pulse rate, but in the dosages usually given does not have much effect on the working or maximum pulse level. For this reason, it does not interfere with a training effect, although allowance must be made for the fact that it can produce a resting bradycardia, which should not be confused with the effects of training.

If You Are Suffering From Skipped Beats

When you take your pulse, you are counting your heart *rate*. At the same time, you are also noting the heart rhythm and how regular it is. The commonest form of irregularity is one in which there appears to be a missed or *skipped* beat. This can be alarming to the novice pulse taker, who may think that the heart has actually dropped a beat or, if the pause is sufficiently long, may imagine that the heart has actually stopped beating. If you realize that one of the medical terms for a skipped beat is a *premature* beat (or extrasystole), you are more likely to be reassured.

Let us take a look at what happens during the cardiac cycle. During the period of systole, blood is ejected into the aorta by the powerful muscular left ventricle. This is felt throughout the arteries of the body as the pulse. During the period of diastole that follows, both right and left ventricles are relaxed, and blood flows back from the body and the lungs through the atria into the ventricles again. If a heart beat occurs prematurely, the period of diastole is shortened, and therefore less blood enters the ventricles. This in turn means that the volume of blood ejected during the following period of systole is also reduced and may not even be sufficient to transmit a palpable impulse to the carotid or radial arteries: thus the "skipped" beat. Nevertheless, the fact that you cannot feel the pulse should not alarm you into thinking that the heart has failed to beat; in fact, the beat has occurred, but earlier than expected.

Why do skipped, or premature, beats occur? A clue to the answer lies in the other medical term for skipped beats. They are also known as *ectopic* beats. Ectopic comes from the Greek meaning "away from the place." The normal signal for a heartbeat originates in a button of specialized tissue (the sinoatrial node) located in the upper corner of the right atrium (Figure 39). From there, 72 times every minute, the signal spreads through the walls of the top

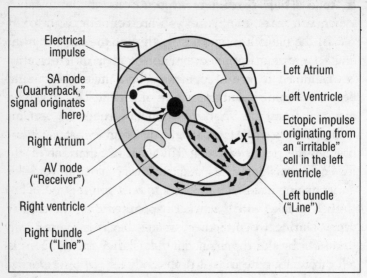

Figure 39: How the Heart Beats
The electrical signal starts in the SA node, passes to the AV node, and then travels along both right and left bundles. An ectopic impulse, causing a premature beat, is also shown.

of the heart to reach a receiver, another collection of specialized cells, situated between the atria and the ventricles at the top of the intraventricular septum (the atrioventricular [AV] node). From the AV node, the signal then proceeds down the intraventricular septum by way of two tracks known as the right and left bundles, and finally ascends the walls of both ventricles. Once its journey is complete, the ventricles contract and the heartbeat occurs. You will remember that the passage of this signal is charted electrically on the electrocardiogram; the P wave represents the start of the message from the SA node (or, if you wish to think of it in football terms, the quarterback) through the atria to the AV node (or receiver) and the QRS deflection marks the completion of the signal (or play) through the bundles (or lines).

Because the heart is such a vital organ, it has a number of built-in safeguards to ensure that it continues to work in spite of any number of malfunctions. If, for instance, our quarterback, the SA node, who is programmed to fire a pass 72 times a minute, is injured, that does not mean that play cannot commence. The AV node, or receiver, is programmed to fire at the rate of 64 times per minute. If, after waiting a suitable period of time, it fails to receive a signal from the SA node, it initiates its own, sending it down both lines to complete the journey as usual and trigger the next heartbeat. But what if our receiver, the AV node, is injured? Is it game over? Not on your life (no pun intended). Heart muscle cells are unique. They are all endowed with the property we refer to as automaticity. It means that, when the need arises, they can automatically take the place of the SA node; that is, they are all potential quarterbacks. The cells in the ventricles are programmed to fire at the rate of 32 beats per minute. If signals are not received from the SA node or the AV node, then, again after waiting an appropriate period of time, they can fire a signal to any part of the right or left bundle below the AV node, set the line in action, and make sure that the ventricles contract. A signal coming from one of these cells originates in an area away from its rightful place, the SA node, and is therefore referred to as being ectopic in origin.

Why do ectopic or premature ventricular beats occur? Some individuals have ventricular muscle heart cells that are overly ambitious to become quarterbacks. These are the "race horse" types. When their adrenaline is flowing, their heart cells are all "fired up," too impatient to await the orderly sequence of play, and so one of them fires off a signal prematurely. Since they are located closer to the conducting bundles than the SA node, their signal arrives first and is often well on its way even before the AV node is activated. Thus the premature beat occurs very shortly after the prior normal beat. At the same time, both SA and AV nodes, recognizing that they have been forestalled, abort their own signals and wait for the next cardiac cycle to start. Because the ectopic beat is premature, there appears to be a longer pause, or skip, occurring before the next normal beat. In fact, the time interval between the normal beat, the premature beat, and the next normal beat is the same as that which would occur between three normal beats. However, because the premature beat is not felt at the pulse, it seems that a very lengthy pause has occurred.

Some individuals' heart cells are susceptible to stimulants such as caffeine (tea, coffee, cola drinks, chocolate), cigarette smoke, excessive alcohol (usually spirits), stressful circumstances that lead to the release of adrenaline and noradrenaline, fatigue, or, in the case of coronary artery disease, shortage of blood supply to the heart muscle. Most people experience isolated skipped beats from time to time, but when they become frequent (every second, third, or fourth beat), are aggravated by physical exertion, and are found in the presence of known coronary artery disease, then they should be reported to the physician before regular exercise training is undertaken. Various techniques for obtaining ambulatory electrocardiogram tracings are now available, and these can often pinpoint the precise source of the ectopic cell. The decision can then be taken as to whether they need to be suppressed by medication or other medical-surgical techniques.

The medical profession has gone through a series of changes of thinking with regard to the treatment of skipped beats. In the First World War, an irregular heartbeat was considered to be a sign of cardiac disease, and if it was detected in the young conscript or draftee, he was labelled with the rather vague diagnosis of D.A.H. (disordered action of the heart) and rejected for service. However, by the Second World War it was recognized that, in the absence of proven heart disease, episodes of irregular heart action were quite common in young men of draft age. Indeed, many of these individuals flew bombers and fighter planes in the Royal Canadian Air Force throughout the war, and a follow-up into their sixties and seventies showed that their subsequent incidence of heart disease was no different from individuals who are free from skipped beats. As the epidemic of coronary disease spread in the postwar period, and with the development of sophisticated electrocardiogram monitoring techniques, once again cardiac irregularities began to be seen in the coronary care units in association with heart attacks. At the same time, new drugs appeared on the scene that were capable of suppressing these extra beats. However, it should be pointed out that these drugs have side effects, and considerable judgment and skill must be exercised by the physician who prescribes them.

In very recent years there has been a tendency to use less drug medication, based on the realization that many types of skipped beats, or arrhythmias as they are known, are not life threatening. In general, they have to be quite frequent and accompanied by symptoms such as blackouts or fainting before being considered for treatment by anti-arrhythmic drugs.

11. Exercise Do's and Don'ts

Don't Expect Miracles

A few basic facts about physical fitness should be borne in mind. First, each of us has an optimal level of endurance fitness appropriate for our age and genetic background. Once we reach that level, more intensive training will result in only marginal gains. Unfortunately, few if any of us even come close to our optimal level. The training tables in Appendix B have been devised to help you achieve a level of fitness that is suitable for your age and general tolerance. They are based on maximum oxygen intake levels attained by patients on our postcoronary exercise program and should, therefore, be well within the capabilities of the vast majority of readers. Of course, there are always exceptions to the rule. For example, some people will be unable to progress to the end of Phase 3. They may stick at an earlier level because of adverse symptoms, failure to achieve the progressing heart rate, or excessive fatigue after the workout. Does this mean that they are wasting their time training? Certainly not. It simply means that they have attained their appropriate duration and intensity of workout, and if they continue to train at this level, they will maintain their optimal fitness.

There is a misapprehension about the development of fitness that is important to dispel. Most people believe that a training program, carried out regularly, results in a gradual day-by-day improvement in their physical state. If you are expecting to progress in this manner, you will be disappointed. What usually happens is that you work away for weeks, or even months, without any apparent change, and then suddenly one day, you find the prescribed training session quite easy. At the same time, you notice that your postworkout pulse rate has dropped a few beats or more. When the same thing happens on the next workout, you will realize that you have suddenly and almost miraculously attained a new level of fitness.

What is the explanation? One of the major effects of training is to open up new blood capillaries in the skeletal muscle tissue so as to transport more oxygen to the working cells. These new capillaries, so small that they can be seen only under a microscope, do not form gradually. They "open up," almost like a budding flower seen under time-lapse photography, in response to the stimulus of repeated and prolonged training sessions. The duration of their formative period varies from individual to individual, but the "plateau" between periods of increased capillarization is an essential part of the process. Don't become discouraged because your condition appears to be stationary. In fact, the preliminary work of capillarization is continuing apace; the next day or week may see the great leap forward.

Do Jog in the Correct Manner
Recreational jogging for fun and fitness is reputed to have started in New Zealand in the 1960s. It was introduced by the world-famous track coach Arthur Lydiard, who believed in long, slow, distance training for his competitive runners, even his half-milers and milers.

Despite its long history, the technique of jogging still is a mystery to some. It differs from running only in its speed of progression. In our context, jogging means running at a pace no quicker than ten minutes per mile (6 minutes per kilometer) or for our coronary patients, 12 minutes per mile (7.5 minutes per kilometer). The action is simple; take short steps, and always land flat-footed. The body should be erect, the shoulders and neck relaxed, and the head held naturally (if you fix your eyes on an imaginary spot about 30 yards (27 meters) ahead, this will give the correct head inclination). The elbows should be bent not quite to a right angle, so that the hands move backwards and forwards easily about the level of the hips; the more you bend your elbows, the shorter the lever made by the arms, and the faster they will swing back and forth. As any sprinter will tell you, pumping your arms vigorously will automatically increase leg speed; so use an easy relaxed arm motion. The short stride and the flat-foot landing will ensure that your center of gravity remains over the leading foot, thus preventing too much of a forward body lean, which is all very well for the competitive middle distance runner, but plays no part in recreational jogging.

Do Buy the Right Equipment

You will need a stopwatch for counting your pulse and also timing your workout. Most models on the market today are relatively cheap and accurate. However, there is not much point in having an accurate stopwatch if you haven't carefully measured the distance you are walking or jogging. If you are working out on the road, you will get an accurate enough reading from a car odometer; I have rarely found these to be misleading — unless, of course, the hot rodder in the family has fitted your sedan with outsize tires!

Shoes are the most important piece of equipment, and you should not attempt to economize here. Just think of the number of times your feet will strike the ground when you are jogging five hours a week, week in, week out. Your feet need to be protected, and it is precisely for this reason that special shoes have been designed for the jogger. Although each manufacturer has individual variations, the following features tend to be common to all. They are quite light, a pair usually weighing less than 2 pounds (1 kilogram). The sole is flexible, but thick enough to absorb shock. The sole is frequently laminated, with layers of sponge rubber for shock absorption and high-density rubber for stability. An arch support is built in, and the inner aspects of the tongue specially padded to protect the instep from the pressure of the laces. The upper is made of nylon, and the portion around the heel (the counter) is reinforced so as to grip the heel firmly and prevent it from wobbling from side to side as you run. Since the heel takes most of our body weight when we run, a special rubber heel wedge is often a feature and, to protect the Achilles tendon, or heel cord, the back of the shoe is reinforced with padding that adds support and prevents chafing.

Needless to say, no one shoe is ideal. Find the particular brand of running shoe that suits you best. In the past 15 years, an incredible number of excellent jogging shoes have appeared on the market, and most sports outfitters will carry an extensive supply. Many of the sales clerks are experts and can help you obtain the right fit and style for your body build and weight.

Do Wear Comfortable Clothes

A *sweat suit* is valuable, but not essential for walking or jogging. A pair of comfortable pants and a sweater will do just as well. Unless you live in Florida or Southern California, much of your training will be done in some form of garb that covers your legs and upper body. A commercial sweat suit is probably the most convenient. My personal preference is for one made from a mixture of nylon and cotton, since it absorbs the sweat much better than a pure nylon suit. Some synthetic materials, such as Goretex, are particularly good at protecting you from the rain or wind. Running shorts and T-shirt complete the list, but neither represents much of a strain on the budget. While some joggers like to avoid socks, the majority prefer a light cotton pair in order to prevent blisters. Vigorously exercising women will want to consider a specially constructed sports bra.

Don't Overtrain

The art of scientific training is to apply just enough overload, or physical stress, to achieve the desired result while at the same time avoiding overstrain and breakdown. Although overtraining is more likely to occur in the competitive athlete than in the fun jogger, nevertheless the coronary-prone individual has a fine margin of error and should recognize the signs and symptoms of excess.

Be alert, therefore, for such signs as excessive muscle soreness, an increase in your resting pulse rate, or undue tiredness persisting to the next training session. Apart from angina, increased palpitations (skipped beats), marked breathlessness, or lightheadedness during an exercise session can also be evidence of shortage of blood to the heart muscle, and their consistent presence during exercise suggests that the coronary blood flow is unable to keep pace with the other training responses. Do not proceed to the next training level if they are present. If they appear for the first time, or become more frequent in response to an exercise prescription, stop your training program and consult your physician.

However, before blaming the prescription entirely for increase in symptoms, consider whether you are under unusual stress at work or are working prolonged hours. Typical postcoronary exercisers are usually enthusiastic and conscientious and often try to maintain the prescribed level of exercise even during busy spells at their job. The result is that when they are at work they worry that they won't have time to carry out their exercise prescription, while during their workout they worry that the time spent in training could have been spent at work. I have learned to beware of various occupations at certain times of the year: for instance, accountants at income tax time, and department store workers during the Christmas season. At these times of stress, the regular exercise prescription may give rise to angina, especially at the end of a long and worrisome day. The obvious solution is to cut back the exercise prescription until the work pattern returns to normal.

If the high stress on the job looks as if it is going to be permanent, you might reduce the level of training. But, in the long run, you would do better to take a serious look at the job itself and your attitude toward it. Are you giving more to your job than your employer expects? Are you trying to carry out a job for which you lack the necessary aptitude? An honest answer to these questions may be very revealing.

Perhaps you should also examine your sleep habits. Chronic lack of sleep seems to be a feature of modern urban living. The long journey home from the office to the suburbs usually means a late evening meal, often followed by watching television until the early hours of the morning (have you noticed how late all the best shows start?). The occasional late night is inevitable, but don't make a habit of it and expect to reap the benefits of training. And don't assume the running program is making you feel overly tired when you haven't bothered to adjust your sleep pattern so as to allow for the additional energy expenditure.

For those who are hooked on exercise, and are jogging five or six miles (8 to 10 kilometers) in an hour, the recognition of overtraining may be difficult. The explanation lies in Dr. Hans Selye's famous theory of stress. The application of mild and healthful stress changes the body's mechanism to make it more resistant to that particular form of stress, and it also produces a feeling of elation and euphoria, which may last for some hours after the stress has been applied. However, if the stress, or in our case, training stimulus, is continued to excessive levels, then specific resistance develops at the cost of generalized resistance. In other words, the highly trained runner becomes extremely resistant to the fatigue of running, but less and less resistant to concurrent infections or mental stress. This is probably the explanation for the high susceptibility of world-class athletes to food poisoning, dysentery, or the sort of flu-like viruses that often rampage through athletes' training camps. In any event, while the loss of generalized resistance may be obvious to a trained observer such as a sports medicine physician or coach, it is often hidden from the athlete by the short-lived sense of well-being that follows each training session. Thus, he or she may be losing weight, becoming more irritable, and developing many of the other symptoms described above; but each time he works out he feels great for two or three hours, and so falls into the trap of repeating the training sessions in the hope that his overall condition will improve. Again, this problem is less common in the fun jogger who is exercising for health, but may be applicable for those who get more seriously involved.

Do Pay Attention to Your Body's Response

In the initial stages of the exercise program, and particularly if you have been sedentary for years, it is inevitable that you will develop mild pain and discomfort in the legs, Achilles tendonitis or inflammation of your heel cord, sore feet, and other relatively minor muscle, tendon, and ligamentous injuries that follow a regimen of walking and jogging after years of inactivity. Although not serious, they are a nuisance and can have an adverse effect on your motivation. A careful warm-up, including stretching, can help, but once again if the problem persists throughout a complete workout, or is felt between the workouts, then a complete rest is indicated. Usually a week is sufficient, but if the trouble recurs on returning to exercise at the end of that time, see your physician, who will probably prescribe a course of physiotherapy. Close adherence to the tables, as well as to the technique of jogging previously described, will reduce such injuries to a minimum. The Toronto Rehabilitation Centre's incidence of injuries over the years has been negligible, despite the fact that we deal almost entirely with middle-aged sedentary individuals who haven't exercised for years.

A pleasant feeling of physical relaxation and tiredness should follow a suitable workout. In many cases, there is an immediate post-exercise sense of exhilaration (for this reason, some people prefer to work out in the morning or early evening rather than just prior to going to bed). Excessive fatigue may be defined as tiredness that is still present after a good night's sleep. It generally responds to three or four days' rest from exercise.

Usually after a workout, the pulse returns to its resting level within two hours; this may take a little longer on a hot and humid day. However, a rapid heart rate (tachycardia) that persists for four hours or longer suggests that the workout has been too intense.

If you find that you are dreading your next workout, this is another sure sign of overtraining. A fit individual usually looks forward to the exercise session, either as a relief from workaday tensions or out of sheer animal spirits. In the early stages of the program, you may not be quite this enthusiastic, but you shouldn't actively dislike the thought of training. If you do, then the exercise prescription is too ambitious and should be reduced.

Don't Continue to Jog If You Suffer from Angina

If you suffer chest pain on exertion, then you should slow your pace until the pain goes away. If the pain does not subside within a hundred yards (91 meters) or so, then stop, and wait for it to disappear. As soon as this happens, start to walk again but at a slower pace. Some individuals can "walk through" their angina, but I caution against this in the early stages of the program until you have become thoroughly familiar with your exercise response.

On occasions, your physician may advise you to take a tablet of nitroglycerine or some similar medication during the workout in order to relieve the angina. Alternatively, you may be asked to take the medication ten minutes or so before your training session in order to prevent the onset of angina. I am frequently asked if this in some way reduces the effectiveness of the training. The answer is no. The fact that it enables you to complete your exercise session is, in itself, proof of its value. As you become more fit, you will find that the angina occurs less and less frequently, until eventually you are able to carry out a full workout without the necessity of medication.

If your angina is so severe that you cannot walk or jog continuously for the prescribed time, don't despair; you can use another training method I have found to be very effective. This is known as interval training; in its modified form, it consists of brisk walking for 15 to 30 seconds at a pace just below that which brings on the chest discomfort. Walk casually for a further minute, and then repeat the brisk walk for another 15 to 30 seconds. In this way, cover a mile (1.6 kilometers), always staying below the level of effort that brings on the pain. You will eventually find that you can extend the distance to 2 or 3 miles (3 to 5 kilometers) in this way, with only infrequent episodes of discomfort.

Don't Exercise after Meals or on an Empty Stomach

Exercise should never be carried out within two hours of eating a heavy meal. This rule is particularly important for angina sufferers, since the digestion of food requires an extra supply of blood to the intestines, thus depleting the coronary circulation. In a situation where the coronary arteries are already narrowed, the loss of even a small reservoir of blood in this area can give rise to myocardial ischaemia.

If you are an early-morning jogger, remember that after eight or ten hours of sleep your blood sugar is very low, and you should not exercise on a completely empty stomach. Have a roll and a glass of orange juice before sallying forth.

Do Warm Up

Angina often occurs during the early part of the workout and can frequently be prevented by a warm-up. This means spending five to ten minutes doing simple calisthenics, or walking at a pace slower than the prescribed intensity, until your body breaks into a light sweat. As soon as the sweat appears, you are then warmed up and may commence your prescription. This is very important for those who suffer from angina and frequently is as effective as taking a nitroglycerine tablet. If your prescription is still at a low level, then you can enhance your warm-up at even slower speeds by wearing a sweater under your track suit to accelerate the onset of the stage of perspiration.

Do Cool Down

Exercise deaths are rare, but when they do occur it is often at the termination of the exercise session, or even on the way to the locker room. Often a careful evaluation of the circumstances will reveal that the unfortunate victim suffered from previously unrecognized coronary disease, had stopped the workout suddenly, and failed to cool down. The suggested mechanism is as follows: Physical effort involves the delivery of a high volume of oxygenated blood to the working muscles and the equally fast return of the deoxygenated blood to the right side of the heart. This return is accelerated by the massaging action of the contracting muscles on their deep veins. If the exerciser stops suddenly, the heart continues to deliver the same volume of blood for the next few seconds, but the pumping action of the muscles ceases, blood pools in the limbs, and there is a sudden drop in the return flow. The result is an equally precipitate drop in the amount of blood ejected in the following heartbeats. Blood pressure falls and coronary blood flow is reduced. This situation in itself can compromise the circulation to the heart muscle.

However, there is further adverse mechanism at work involving changes in the "fight or flight" stress hormones, adrenaline and noradrenaline. Both of these substances, particularly the latter, circulate throughout the body in high concentrations during physical exercise, ensuring that blood pressure and heart rate keep pace with the demand of the working muscles for an enhanced blood supply. With sudden cessation of exercise and blood pooling, the consequent sharp drop in blood pressure is interpreted by the brain as a failure in the blood delivery system, with the result that there is an immediate release of even greater quantities of noradrenaline in order to correct the situation. From animal studies, we know that if we suddenly expose atherosclerotic hearts to abnormally high concentrations of noradrenaline, we frequently induce cardiac arrest. The lesson, then, is obvious. Spend five or ten minutes winding down after your exercise session, moving around and gradually letting your body return to its resting level.

While on the topic, a caution should be sounded against having hot showers immediately after a workout. A significant proportion of blood flow has already been diverted to the muscles. A hot shower dilates the blood vessels of the skin, further reducing the flow through the coronary circulation. This situation, following an exercise session, may prove too much for the individual with coronary artery disease. So I advise all my patients to wait 10 or 15 minutes after exercising before taking a lukewarm shower.

Do Choose a Flat Course

Hill running may be great training for competitive athletes, but it should be avoided by middle-aged joggers. It will certainly aggravate a tendency to angina, since the energy expended in running up a slope can be considerable. All of the distances listed in the tables are assumed to be on a flat course. Ideally, therefore, all of your workouts should be on the flat. If hills are unavoidable, then reduce your speed accordingly so as to achieve the same heart rate and/ or rating of perceived exertion on the Borg scale you associate with your usual course.

Do Beware Summer Heat

Your body temperature results from a combination of heat generated by your working muscles and internal organs and heat absorbed from the surrounding air. As you sit reading this book, presumably relaxed and calm, you are generating about 75 calories of heat every hour. If you were to put the book down (not yet, please), stand up and go for a 3-mile (5-kilometer) walk, you would generate about 300 calories an hour.

If the body had no means of dissipating its internal heat, then even under the resting conditions, your temperature would rise about 2°F (1°C) an hour; under moderate working conditions, the rise would be in the order of 9°F (5°C) an hour. Like any other machine, the body has a temperature at which all the various parts function most efficiently, 98.6°F (37°C). If the temperature of the body climbs above 110°F (43°C) or falls below 84°F (29°C), essential organs such as the heart, kidneys, and liver cease to work, and death becomes imminent. But since, as we have seen, even staying alive generates enough heat to kill us in a matter of hours, we must have a very efficient mechanism for dissipating this excess heat and holding the body temperature consistently close to the 98.6°F (37°C) level. How does this system work?

Physical exercise results in the shunting of as much as a gallon (3.8 liters) of blood through the blood vessels of the muscles every minute. Since these muscles are working, their internal temperature is raised, and this heats the blood that passes through them. The heated blood then returns to the heart, where it is pumped around the body again. As it flows through the brain, it triggers off the Benzinger Reflex, a mechanism by which the blood vessels to the skin are opened up and the sweat glands stimulated to work overtime. Warm blood can now dissipate its heat into the surrounding *cooler* air by the processes of convection, conduction, and radiation. Notice I said *cooler* air — that is, an air temperature lower than the skin temperature of 92°F (33°C). What happens when the air temperature is high, approaching that of the skin? Under these circumstances, the body has to depend more and more on the evaporation of sweat to lower the body temperature. The mere act of sweating has no cooling effect per se; it is the vaporization, or evaporation of the sweat from the surface of the body that is all important.

There is a limit to the rate at which one can sweat. In the average unconditioned individual this amounts to about 1 quart (1 liter) per hour; in a trained heat-acclimatized exerciser, this figure may be increased to as much as 1 gallon (3.8 liters) per hour. Evaporation of sweat can also be influenced by a number of physical conditions. If the air is humid, it is already saturated with moisture and cannot accept any more. So the sweat will not vaporize; it will merely drip down the face and body and exert no cooling effect. In conditions of very high humidity, therefore, sweating becomes ineffective as a means of reducing body temperature.

On a windy day, the process of evaporation has an advantage. The air next to the sweating skin, as soon as it becomes heavily laden with sweat moisture, is blown away, and its place is taken by air that is drier and more receptive to further evaporation.

Clothing is an important factor. It should allow free movement of air over the skin. Trapped pockets of air become saturated with vaporized sweat and prevent further evaporation from that area. Air is a very good insulator and prevents body heat from escaping by conduction or radiation. Examples of clothing that prevent adequate heat loss are the rubberized training suit, or the footballer's uniform, with its plastic helmet and padding, designed to protect against bodily contact injury but not against the ill effects of high heat conditions. Deaths from heatstroke due to the wearing of such apparel are, sad to say, recorded from time to time in the medical literature.

A further condition affecting sweat evaporation has to do with blood volume. On a hot day when exercising, you sweat heavily and lose water from your blood at the rate of 2.5 quarts (2.5 liters) per hour. Unless you replace the sweat loss by drinking fluids, the net result will be a reduction in blood volume. But as long as you keep jogging, your muscles require oxygen and thus your heart is committed to pumping a steady supply of oxygen-laden blood to the scene of action. With the drop in the amount of blood available, however, there is a drop in the amount ejected with each heartbeat. The only way that the heart can now maintain its output of blood is to increase the number of strokes per minute. In other words, the heart rate must go up if the heart is to maintain an adequate blood supply to the exercising muscles.

If you continue to exercise at the same intensity, your maximum heart rate is eventually reached. When that happens, cardiac output cannot keep pace with demand. Actually, you can gain a very slight respite by constricting the blood vessels of the skin, a stratagem that shunts some blood back into the central pool, raising the central blood volume, and once more makes blood available for the heart to pump. Unfortunately, the price you have paid for this temporary postponement of the inevitable is a high one. By diverting blood away from the skin, you have deprived yourself of your major mechanism of heat loss. Thus the temperature inside your body rapidly begins to climb, and the whole heat-control compensatory system begins to break down. Unless you stop exercising, or unless you have been drinking ample quantities of fluid to replenish your blood volume, you have reached the stage of dehydration.

There are three clinical conditions associated with exercising in the hot weather. Although they may merge imperceptibly and insidiously into one another, to understand the whole mechanism of dehydration let us deal with them as separate entities.

Heat Cramps

Heat cramps occur in highly trained individuals who are working for an hour or more in hot weather. They may come on toward the end of an exercise session or after it, for example, in the shower. They can be extremely severe and may last for many minutes.

Such cramps are thought to be due to a chronic lack or loss of sodium. As I explained earlier, the highly conditioned athlete has a copious sweat production, much greater than the sedentary individual. While the sweat contains less sodium than normal (the body's attempt to conserve its supply), this can be outbalanced by the speed with which sweating occurs, so that eventually there is a tendency to lose sodium. Over the short term, the fluid can be replaced by drinking water, but this does not replace sodium. Ingestion of a dilute salt solution (one teaspoonful of salt to one quart, or 5 milliliters of salt to 1 liter) will relieve the cramps very rapidly.

The average walker or jogger is not likely to be bothered by these heat cramps. They are much more frequent in the individual who is training for long periods in the heat. Incidentally, your best sources of salt are catsup, bran, fish, nuts, and meat. Do not use salt tablets; they are far too concentrated a source.

Heat Exhaustion

This condition results from an inadequate replacement of the water lost in sweat. The early signs are fatigue and weakness. I cannot emphasize enough that thirst is a very poor indicator that you need fluid. The mere act of putting something in the mouth, a pebble, for instance, reduces the sensation of thirst for about 15 minutes. Laboratory experiments have shown that the introduction of a small amount of fluid through a tube directly into the stomach has the same effect — even though the water has not been absorbed through the stomach wall. So you may take just a mouthful of cold water, swallow it, no longer feel thirsty, and carry on exercising for another half an hour before you feel the need to drink again, yet the amount of fluid taken is totally inadequate.

With water losses of up to 5% of body weight, the dehydrated exerciser develops a flushed, hot skin, judgment becomes poor, movement is uncoordinated and behavior irrational. Other symptoms of heat exhaustion are light-headedness, a very rapid heart rate, and severe frontal headaches. Heat exhaustion can occur in varying degrees of severity and may become chronic during a long spell of hot-weather training. Drinking adequate water before, during, and after training walks or jogs is just as important as during a football game or a marathon run. Heat exhaustion can also develop rapidly during exercise and may progress to heatstroke, the third and most dangerous manifestation of dehydration.

Heatstroke

Heatstroke is the popular term for hyperpyrexia, that is, body temperature in excess of 108°F (42°C). Again, the cause is lack of water. Its onset can be insidious and rapid. The victims, after demonstrating evidence of extreme heat exhaustion, collapse into a coma, from which they may never recover. Death is frequently due to kidney failure.

The effects of heatstroke on the body are widespread. In the posterior portion of the brain, the cerebellum, there is destruction of specialized cells. For this reason, survivors may be left with staggering gait, or speech disorders. Bleeding into the cortex of the brain is responsible for various mental disturbances. The kidneys can be irreparably damaged, making renal dialysis necessary. Hemorrhage into the heart muscle, and even heart attacks in spite of perfectly normal coronary arteries, have been reported. Clotting of blood in the blood vessels may lead to damage in a whole host of organs. As you can see, an incredible number of deadly pathological changes all stem from simple failure to drink adequately during hot-weather exercise.

How to Avoid Dehydration

Anyone who exercises on a hot day, old or young, male or female, walker, jogger, or runner, is a potential dehydration victim. If you are fun jogger, never forget that the number of calories burned (and therefore the amount of body heat generated) doesn't depend on the speed you jog, but rather on the distance you cover. For example, whether you jog 3 miles (5 kilometers) in 24 minutes or in 36, you will still burn approximately the same number of calories. Remember that if you are a long-distance walker, the slower the pace, the longer you are exposed to the sun, and so the greater the likelihood of dehydration.

The ratio of your body weight to your surface area (W/SA ratio) is an important factor in your ability to cope with heat. The larger your surface area, the more you can lose heat to the surrounding air. On the other hand, the greater your muscle mass, the more heat you generate when exercising. If you have a high W/SA ratio (short, muscular stature), then you have difficulty coping with hot-weather exercise. You will produce lots of heat, but will be unable to dissipate it rapidly. On the other hand, if you have a low W/SA ratio (tall, slim build), you will have fewer problems during your summer exercise sessions.

The following rules apply equally to middle-aged novice exercisers, joggers, and walkers of all sizes, and highly trained athletes:

1. Allow time for heat acclimatization. The body learns to cope with heat if you give it enough time to adjust. The process takes about seven to ten days, and during this time, the workouts should be low key to commence with, gradually building up to your usual intensity and duration.

   The benefits of acclimatization were all too apparent during the Desert Storm Campaign, where one of the U.S. military's greatest concerns was the problem of dehydration. Troops from the hotter areas of the country had many fewer problems with heatstroke and related conditions during training than those from colder states.

   When the temperature is above 86°F (30°C) and the humidity above 30%, the cardiac exerciser should miss the workout altogether. If in doubt, consult Appendix C for use of the Heat Safety Index.

2. Always prehydrate 10 to 20 minutes or so before exercising on a warm day. Drink about 1 cup (250 milliliters) of fluid, then another 1 cup every 20 minutes or so while working out. Don't wait to feel thirsty before drinking.

3. The best fluid to use is water. It should be comfortably cold (best temperature for absorption is about 40°F (4.4°C), and if you require a flavor you may add a little fruit juice according to taste. Minerals such as sodium and potassium aren't really essential; the body can replace them later. However, if you do add sodium, it should be in small amounts of 1 teaspoon (5 milliliters) of salt to 1 gallon (3.8 liters) of water.

4. Some postcoronary exercisers may be taking hydro-chlorothiazide medication, a diuretic that is given to treat mild cases of high blood pressure. Diuretics encourage the kidneys to excrete sodium and, therefore, water. Potassium is lost in the urine at the same time, and the prescribing physician often suggests that a patient on such medication increase his or her consumption of potassium-containing foods or, alternatively, pre-scribes a potassium pill. Obviously, a patient taking diuretics (trade names, Diuril, HydroDiuril, Esiberix) is most susceptible to low blood potassium levels in high-heat training and should be aware of this. Too much or too little potassium in the blood can give rise to various abnormalities of cardiac rhythm. In unexplained cases of palpitations or skipped beats appearing in a healthy exerciser, analysis of blood sample for potassium concentrations should be carried out.

Other medications that may affect tolerance to heat are beta-blockers. They reduce the rate of sweating and so may predispose to heat stress. Alcohol acts as a diuretic and so should be avoided before exercise. Furthermore, it impairs judgment and may encourage ill-advised overexertion.

Sugar, usually in the form of glucose, is often added to replacement fluid to provide energy. Actually, there is little to recommend this practice. Glucose solutions that exceed 2.5% strength are too concentrated to be absorbed through the gut wall and therefore lie in the stomach, causing nausea and vomiting. Worse still, to dilute the glucose, water is actually drawn out of the bloodstream and cells of the body into the intestine, thus aggravating the dehydration! If, on the other hand, you prepare a solution containing less than 2.5% glucose, the amount of energy provided is probably too small to be of any value.

The best replacement fluid, then, is still cold water, plus a mild flavoring agent if desired.

5. Clothing should be light, porous, and comfortable. Fishnet vests are most suitable, allowing easy circulation of air and free evaporation of sweat from the skin.

6. Cold water sponging helps, as will putting ice under your hat. If you sponge your legs, be careful not to wet your shoes and socks, otherwise you may develop blisters.

7. Get into the habit of weighing yourself naked before and after each workout. If you have hydrated adequately, you should have lost no more than 3% of your body weight; more than 5%, and you have definitely dehydrated.

8. Finally, when the air temperature and humidity are both extremely high even copious quantities of water will not hold your body temperature down. Slowing your pace, or even walking, will reduce your body's rate of heat generation, but if you start to develop symptoms of excessive body temperature (muscle and abdominal cramps, dizziness, a tendency to stumble), then smarten up and quit exercising. Failure to do so may have very unpleasant consequences.

Do Be Careful in Cold Weather

While indoor exercising has its advocates, I believe that walking and jogging out-of-doors has much to recommend it. Apart from the sheer boredom and discomfort of indoor exercising (when did you last sweat your way round 4 miles [6.5 kilometers] of a "26-laps-to-the-mile" track?), the out-door exerciser achieves an exhilaration and sense of satisfaction that can be obtained only by physically coping with the natural elements. Besides, if you are going to work out five days a week for the rest of your life, surely the most convenient way to do so is by stepping through your front door and using your own district as a training ground. You fit your exercising into your lifestyle, and you make it part of your daily living.

There are, of course, some hazards associated with exercising in the cold. There is no doubt that the body's reaction to cold puts a stress on the cardiovascular system. When the body temperature falls, it tries to conserve heat by constricting the blood vessels in the skin. This action shunts the warm blood away from the surface and reduces heat loss from conduction, convection, and radiation. The cost of this sudden narrowing of a major portion of the blood vessel system is a rapid rise in the pressure against which the heart is pumping — in other words, a rise in blood pressure. The additional load on the heart brought about by the increase in Rate Pressure Product (HR × BP) may be sufficient to induce angina in an individual with narrowed coronary arteries.

How is it, though, that tens of thousands of people, from the young to the elderly, can walk, jog, cross-country ski, and skate, with considerable exhilaration and pleasure, despite freezing temperatures? The answer is that the body heat generated by physical activity balances the heat lost to the surrounding air. Skin temperature is therefore maintained at about 92°F (33°C) and a comfortable equi- librium is reached. Cold-induced constriction of skin blood vessels does not occur, and there is no increase in the work load placed upon the heart. However, of the two variables (heat loss and heat production), the ability to generate adequate body heat from exercise may be the most difficult for the person with coronary artery disease. If physical effort is difficult because of angina, then heat loss may exceed heat production, and the chain of events just described is set in motion.

In practice, however, cold-weather angina may be avoided in patients with coronary artery disease. Wearing three or four layers of suitable light clothing increases heat-retaining properties without adding to energy expenditure. For instance, an additional energy expenditure of only four or five calories per minute (for example, walking 1 mile in 15 minutes, or 1 kilometer in 9 minutes), can be accomplished in temperatures even as low as 14°F (−10°C) when you are suitably clothed. Those who develop angina in cold weather even when walking very slowly should exercise outdoors only in warmer weather until training results in a drop in Rate Pressure Product and, thus, angina, for a given level of effort. Eventually, they will be able to exercise in colder temperatures.

Some patients who are capable of higher effort levels still suffer angina within a minute or so of beginning their exercise in the cold. The mechanism responsible is probably reflex coronary vasoconstriction. During exercise, as respiratory rate increases, mouth breathing becomes easier. The warming effect of the blood vessels in the mucous membrane of the nose is bypassed, and cold air stimulates the nerve endings at the back of the throat. This in turn leads to spasm of the coronary arteries. Careful indoor warmup exercise and the use of a woolen scarf covering the mouth may help. In 1968, the Toronto Rehabilitation Centre devised a simple plastic disposable oxygen mask attached to 12 inches (30 centimeters) of flexible tubing extending to beneath the subject's T-shirt to about the level of the chest bone. At a cost of about $10, this easily produced apparatus is highly effective in preventing early-onset cold-induced angina. (It is, incidentally, also effective for patients with emphysema.)

In addition to the possibility of cold-induced angina, we have the problem of snow-covered and icy surfaces, which impose greater energy expenditure and increase the likelihood of injury. Head winds increase chilling effect and air resistance. Rain or wet snow reduces the insulating properties of clothing and allows body heat to "wick out" to the atmosphere. Paradoxically, dehydration can be as much of a problem in the winter as it is in the summer. The evaporative process continues, making excessive fluid loss by sweating possible. Moreover, exposure to cold air strongly suppresses the sense of thirst, and drinking to replace fluid is often ignored.

Fortunately, the body heat generated by fast walking or jogging is usually sufficient to offset loss of heat to the surrounding cold air. Where there is imbalance in favor of heat loss, this can be prevented by wearing suitable clothing.

The purpose of clothing in cold weather is to insulate the surface of the skin from the surrounding environment and prevent heat loss. Clothing traps air and modifies the skin's so-called microclimate. The fabric is less important in this regard than the weave. Layering garments and varying the closeness of the weave or knit allows considerable flexibility in achieving the desired level of heat retention. However, insulating properties may be changed drastically by the action of water or sweat. Tightly woven cotton with little interfiber air-trapping sticks to the body when wet, eliminates large air pockets, and reduces insulation. Wool, on the other hand, retains its insulating properties with its natural oils and greater air-trapping interstices even when wet. In recent years, synthetic fibers have been woven and knit in various ways to develop systems of functional clothing for cold weather activities of all types.

The layer next to the skin should be tightly woven ribbed material that provides some insulation while allowing for evaporation during excessive sweating. The middle layer (loosely woven wool or a fishnet cotton and synthetic mix) should absorb some of this excess sweat but again allow for evaporation. The third layer (a tighter woven wool, wool/cotton combination, or synthetic fiber) should have some degree of stretch to permit variable insulation by opening and closing the weave in the material in response to body movement. A fourth layer is needed only in conditions of high wind and extreme cold. It should protect against wind, rain, and snow and yet be permeable to body heat. Synthetic materials have performed these functions with considerable success.

If possible, all upper body garments should be zipped or buttoned in such a way that they can be loosened at the neck when the body overheats or closed up if chilling occurs. Dark or colored outer garments tend to conserve body heat; they should be adorned with reflective strip material so as to be visible in the darkness.

The legs rarely require more than two layers. Track suit pants over pantihose will suffice on even the coldest days. Long underwear is fine, although it tends to restrict knee movement unless it is cut down to shorts length. Socks should be a wool/cotton mixture or a ribbed and channelled, woven synthetic material. Hands, susceptible to cold because they are poorly muscled and used little in jogging, are best protected by wool mittens, which trap more air than gloves. Since considerable body heat is lost through the head, a woolen hat that pulls down over the ears to prevent frostbite is necessary: on very cold days a balaclava, which leaves only the eyes, nose, and mouth exposed, is a good idea. The exposed parts of the face should be protected from chapping and cold sores by applying petroleum jelly. Shoes with waffle soles give greater purchase on ice.

Air temperature is only one of the factors that should be taken into consideration when planning workouts in cold climates. Wind conditions, presence or absence of sunshine, and humidity all affect the body cooling rate.

A 15-mile-an-hour (24-kilometer-an-hour) wind can make a still-air temperature reading of 36°F (2°C) feel like 16°F (−9°C); thus a wind chill chart should always be consulted on a windy day (see Appendix D).

Is the sun shining or is it overcast? Direct sunshine is worth an additional 13°F (7°C). This can be critical. You may start your walk on a calm day with the sun shining brightly, and if you are using an out-and-back course, by the time you head for home you may find yourself battling a 10-mile-an-hour (16-kilometer-an-hour) wind, with the sun long since disappeared behind the clouds. You are no longer adequately dressed, and things soon become pretty miserable. You can, of course, pick up your pace to generate more body heat. But this may require a level of exertion beyond your capabilities, in which case you will fatigue, lose your body heat even more rapidly or, if you are a postcoronary patient, develop angina and have to slow down again.

Probably the greatest threat to maintaining equilibrium between heat production and heat loss is wet clothing. Whether the cause is driving rain, melting snow, or drenching perspiration, the effect is the same. Evaporation from the wet material will drop your body temperature at an alarming rate. This is one of the most potent causes of hypothermia. With every two degrees Fahrenheit (one degree Celsius) fall below normal, you go through the successive stages of slurred speech, uncoordination of hands and feet, unsteadiness, confusion, collapse, and finally coma. Hypothermia is hardly the lot of everyone who goes for a walk or jog on a cold day and gets their clothes wet, but you should take precautions to see that you never put yourself in the position of risking such a tragedy.

Putting all of this together, we can lay down the following guidelines for cold-weather exercising:

1. Wear layers of clothing that are woven to regulate heat loss.
2. Always consult the wind chill chart (see Appendix D) on windy days and use the effective temperature rather than the air temperature as a guideline. If the effective temperature is below 14°F (−10°C), postcoronary exercisers should question the wisdom of exercising out of doors.

3. Because the wind and sun conditions can change rapidly, a short out-and-back course should be chosen, the furthest point of which should be no more than a quarter of a mile (half a kilometer) from the starting point. This is particularly important for the less fit.

4. In wet and cold conditions, the clothing layers should include a light cotton and nylon mixture outer garment that will provide two to three hours of protection against moisture.

5. Head winds must be taken into consideration and the pace adjusted downward to maintain the prescribed level of energy expenditure. If one does not reduce pace in the teeth of a head wind, then premature fatigue will inevitably ensue, a slower pace will lead to inadequate heat production, and symptoms from chilling will occur.

    By how much should the pace be slowed? Pulse rate during normal workout conditions may be used as a guideline. Alternatively, back off the pace until you are experiencing the same level of breathing rate and leg muscle exertion you usually associate with your customary exercise pace, generally 12 or 13 on the numerical Borg Scale of Perceived Exertion (page 191). This will correlate with the heart rate, blood pressure, and oxygen intake associated with your usual workout, even though, because of difficult or adverse conditions such as head winds or hilly terrain, the speed of the walk/jog is necessarily slower. I find this is true for many of my patients, but it does cause problems in those "deniers" who consistently overestimate their prowess. It can also be a dangerous rule of thumb for patients who develop increased skipped beats with exercise and who can detect them only by pulse taking.

6. Frostbite is unusual in the walker/jogger, but can occur in poorly protected hands, ears, and faces exposed to temperatures below 30°F (−1°C). Failure to take wind chill into account is usually the cause.

For more than 25 winters, a high percentage of some 12,000 patients on the Toronto program have trained outdoors on all but the severest days without ill effects. They are the finest testimonial to our approach. The trouble is, by the time winter has come to an end, they have to start acclimatizing to the heat again. Such is life!

Don't Do Heavy Isometric Exercises

A maximum isometric muscle contraction is one in which the muscle contracts with full force but without shortening. For example, normally, when the biceps muscle in your upper arm contracts, your elbow bends. If you contract the muscle while at the same time holding the elbow joint rigid, you have achieved an isometric contraction of your biceps. Examples of isometric effort in everyday life are straining to raise a jammed window, trying to lift a too-heavy suitcase, or attempting to push a snow-bound automobile. This type of muscle action, as opposed to the "isotonic" movement in which the joint is allowed to move and the muscle to shorten, causes a sharp rise in the diastolic blood pressure and a marked increase in the pressures within the chambers of the heart. If the heart wall is scarred from a previous heart attack, and if the coronary blood circulation is impaired as a result of atherosclerosis, then the results of such pressure increases can be dangerous. Lifting of heavy weights is, for this reason, prohibited as a training endeavor or a recreational sport for heart patients. Straining to lift heavier and heavier loads may well build the body beautiful, but the isometric element involved makes it an avocation suitable only for those with the healthiest of cardiovascular systems.

An example of the adverse cardiovascular effects of an isometric effort is found in Lord Moran's book on Sir Winston Churchill:

Washington, December 17. "I am glad you have come," the P.M. began. He was in bed and looked worried. "It was hot last night, and I got up to open the window. It was very stiff. I had to use considerable force and I noticed all at once I was short of breath. I had a dull pain over my heart. It went down my left arm. It did not last very long, but it has never happened before. What is it? Is my heart all right? I thought of sending for you, but it passed off."

Sir Winston was an astute observer of symptoms. He was describing typical angina pectoris as the result of an excessive load on his heart and coronary vasculature.

An additional problem with all isometric exercises is that the uninitiated tend to hold their breath while carrying them out. While this may seem to enhance performance, it introduces another element of danger for the person with heart problems. A not uncommon sight in any gymnasium is an exerciser slowly going blue in the face as he attempts to strain himself to the limit. By holding his breath, he has closed off his windpipe, and in the course of his exercise is forcing the air into his lungs against the closed valve. This state of affairs is referred to in physiological circles as the Valsalva maneuver. Its effect, like that of the isometric muscle contraction, is to throw a heavy burden on a heart already severely taxed by the particular exercise that is being carried out. Hence power calisthenics, or any physical activity that encourages the Valsalva maneuver, is off limits for the individual at risk.

Do Take Care When Shovelling Snow

The incidence of fatal heart attack and sudden cardiac death in any large city inevitably mounts in the three or four days after a heavy snowstorm. These deaths are almost entirely the result of snow shovelling, which has particularly adverse effects on the elderly and those with coronary artery disease. The activity has all the components necessary to put the cardiovascular system in jeopardy. It is not only a very intense form of exercise, equivalent to running a mile (1.6 kilometers) at anywhere between 7 and 12 minutes (depending on whether you are moving heavy wet or dry light snow); it is also usually performed under unfavorable conditions of extreme cold. Add to that the most dangerous element of all — the repeated isometric arm contractions, customarily accompanied by the Valsalva maneuver, and you have set the stage for potential disaster.

If you have to move snow, do it as follows. Dress for the cold in the manner advised under the section on "Cold Weather Exercise" earlier in this chapter, and always warm up for four or five minutes before starting. Push the snow with a scoop rather than lifting it with a shovel; this action allows your legs to do the work isotonically rather than your arms isometrically. Take a rest every three minutes or so and don't let yourself get out of breath. If you suffer from angina, or have severe coronary artery disease, give the chore to someone else, and have a hot drink ready for them when they finish.

Does this mean that you must be in constant fear of holding your breath or inadvertently carrying out an isometric muscle contraction? Of course not. As a matter of fact, the more endurance fitness you develop, the stronger your heart, and the more it will be able to resist such stresses and strains. My point is that you should be aware of the dangers of these types of exertions, should not practice them on a regular basis, and certainly should not include them as part of your training program.

Do Beware of Saunas and Steam Baths

Postcoronary patients have been found to develop electro cardiographic evidence of myocardial ischaemia while in the sauna; these changes took the form of ST segment depression and frequent ectopic beats. They did not occur to anything like the same extent when these same subjects exercised to a heart rate level equivalent to that attained in the sauna. The reason for this is that excessive heat, like emotional stress, releases large quantities of noradrenaline and adrenaline into the bloodstream, which may have adverse effects on the myocardium. Potentially dangerous falls in blood pressure levels have been reported as a result of dilation of skin vessels (especially when the subject is in the sitting position) with resultant decrease in coronary blood flow.

Steam baths, whirlpools, and hot tubs utilize moist heat, which is the least well tolerated by the body, since it prevents loss of heat by evaporation, or sweating, and permits the body temperature to rise more quickly to sometimes dangerous levels. Saunas, on the other hand, because they use dry heat, permit sweating, but are often very hot, 170°F (77°C), or more. The excessive sweating can cause dehydration. The loss of water from the blood makes the blood thicker and more likely to clot inside an atherosclerotic coronary, and possibly cause a heart attack.

If you use the sauna, drink plenty of water to replace that lost in the sweat. Choose a cooler type of bath, or limit the stay in higher temperatures to five minutes. Do not use the steam bath to "sweat out" symptoms that might well be the early warning of coronary artery disease (for example, "muscular" chest pain, excessive fatigue, or "bursitis" in the shoulder). Above all, do not, out of a false sense of pride, attempt to "tough it out" if you feel yourself getting dizzy, breathless, or developing an unpleasant thumping of your heart.

Don't Exercise When Pollution Levels Are High

What are the common air pollutants? What effect do they have on us? The answer to the first question depends on the area in which you live. In Los Angeles, for instance, the pollutants are composed largely of compounds that arise from the chemical interaction between sunlight and the various combustible products of automobile fumes. In other cities, we may be dealing predominantly with carbon monoxide, sulphur dioxide, or a number of airborne chemicals in particulate form.

Carbon monoxide is a major component of cigarette smoke, and we have already described its cuckoo-like occupancy of the red cells of the blood, displacing the vital oxygen being carried to the body's cells. Inhaled even in minute quantities by the exerciser, it could reduce the efficiency of their oxygen transport system and turn an easy workout into a relatively tough one. Inhaling enough carbon monoxide to affect about 20% of the hemoglobin, the oxygen-carrying protein in the blood, will lead to headache behind and over the eyes, breathlessness, muscular weakness, and dizziness. When about 40% of the available hemoglobin is saturated with carbon monoxide, there is a feeling of nausea, severe headache, and breathlessness on exertion, together with dimming and blurring of vision; judgment becomes impaired and the individual becomes belligerent; there is lack of coordination, stumbling, and possibly even collapse. Some studies have shown that patients with coronary heart disease can develop angina or electrocardiographic evidence of myocardial ischaemic changes with carbon monoxide levels as low as 3% to 5%. Thus, since the major source of carbon monoxide is from automobile exhaust fumes, you should avoid walking or jogging close to heavily traveled main streets or highways. Exhaust smoke, however, disperses slowly, so if your jogging route is 40 to 60 feet (12 to 18 meters) or more away from the edge of a busy highway, you should reduce the risk; better still, try to find a route through a park, green belt, or a relatively smog-free suburb.

Ozone is a key component in the smog that results from the action of sunlight on fuel-oil hydrocarbons and nitrogen dioxide. It has been found in aircraft cabins at altitudes above 30,000 feet, and also in association with various welding devices. In recent years, a good deal of work has been carried out on the effect of ozone on the human body, and while much is still to be learned, we do have some indications that in high concentrations (greater than 0.15 parts per million of air), it can have some toxic effect. Its major target is the respiratory organs, where it can cause breathlessness, chest pain, and coughing. In addition to the respiratory symptoms, high ozone levels can cause headaches and reduce one's ability to concentrate. The heart rate may decrease, and this can give rise to increases in blood carbon dioxide. At ozone levels in excess of 0.2 parts per million, there may be a considerable decrease in central visual acuity and ability to see in the dark. Some coaches have reported that when the ozone levels are high, athletic performance is adversely affected.

A few cities now operate an ozone alert when the level reaches more than 0.15 parts per million, which warns susceptible individuals to reduce physical exertion. When the level becomes in excess of 0.2 parts per million, even healthy persons should limit their outdoor exercise. It is possible, however, to defeat the ozone problem if you remember one or two basic principles. In the first place, keep in mind that on a sunny, humid day the maximal ozone levels occur between 11:00 a.m. and 6:00 p.m., and the lowest levels occur in the early morning. Therefore, if you wish to be on the safe side, exercise early in the morning or late at night. Older individuals (and that means us) are more susceptible to the effects of ozone than young people. Don't forget that the hotter it gets, the more ozone is produced. Secondly, if you have a chest infection, you are obviously more susceptible. Interestingly, the ingestion of Vitamin C would appear to substantially reduce the effect of ozone on the lungs. Finally (and this must be a consolation to Los Angeleans), the more exposure you have to ozone, the more likely you are to develop a tolerance toward it. At least you are less likely to be overcome by the more acute and unpleasant symptoms.

There is no doubt that running in the city on a hot, humid, muggy day when the traffic is heavy and the industrial pall is hanging close to the ground can be uncomfortable and sometimes downright unpleasant. Nevertheless, if you follow these simple guidelines you should not come to any harm, and the benefits of jogging will far outweigh any minor and transitory discomforts brought about by breathing polluted air.

Don't Exercise with a Fever

A number of viral-type infections can involve the heart muscle. The effect may be transitory, lasting only a matter of days or weeks. They may pass unnoticed by the patient and leave no permanent damage. However, strenuous physical activity should be avoided during this time. Although severe viral myocarditis is relatively rare, mild forms of the condition may exist much more frequently than we suspect. Since a visit to the cardiologist is hardly justified every time you develop a fever, be safe rather than sorry: don't exercise if you are suffering from any flu-like illness. To be further on the safe side, you should not work out until a full seven days have elapsed after your temperature has returned to normal.

Don't Abuse Alcohol

Excessive alcohol intake can contribute to obesity and hypertension. Alcohol is a major health problem in many countries today. On the other hand, a number of studies have suggested that light to moderate drinking is associated with a lower incidence of heart attacks than in non-drinking or heavy drinking. The reason seems to be that alcohol in moderation raises HDL-cholesterol. There is also some suggestion that it may lower LDL-cholesterol and also prevent excessive blood clotting. The upper limit of moderate drinking is defined as being no more than two drinks a day.

Having said that, I should emphasize that it is very easy to exceed the "moderate" level. In the patient with coronary disease, alcohol can also depress heart function. The amount of alcohol needed to cause this adverse effect in heart patients is quite small: in one study, just 2 ounces (60 milliliters) of whisky. The heart muscle cells may also suffer permanent damage from prolonged and excessive alcohol consumption. Another practical consideration is body weight. Alcoholic beverages are high in caloric value, so you can scarcely expect to lose weight on a diet of cottage cheese, lettuce, and beer!

For all of the above reasons, consider carefully whether or not to consume alcohol. If you have serious cardiac problems, you are better off abstaining. Chances are, however, that if you are capable of exercising, you are capable of drinking, but in moderation.

Just as you shouldn't drink and drive, so you should never drink before jogging, especially if you suffer from heart disease. Not only is your heart less likely to be able to cope with the additional stress, but your judgment of pace and distance is probably impaired, as is your ability to count your pulse and interpret such warning signs as angina or lightheadedness. If you do drink, then do so in moderation, and *after* your workout.

Do Check the Physical Conditions

Don't underestimate the effect of running into a head wind. It has been shown that an athlete weighing 134 pounds (61 kilograms) and running at a six-minute-mile (3.75-minute-kilometer) pace on a still day expends approximately 6% more oxygen in the face of a light, 10 mph (16 km/hr) wind; to put it another way, he will have to put out the effort of a sub-five-minute-mile (sub-three-minute-kilometer) pace! At 40 mph (64 km/hr), wind increases the oxygen cost by over 40%. When you are talking oxygen increments of that order, you may be getting into a situation that is beyond your maximal oxygen intake. The trick is to back off if you notice yourself getting unusually breathless and tired on a windy day. Allowing for the wind resistance, the slower time will be giving you the same training effect anyway.

The best surface to run on is a smooth one. The hardness or softness doesn't really matter; your shoes should take care of that factor. An uneven surface considerably increases the effort of running, driving up your oxygen intake and heart rate accordingly, and sometimes giving rise to anginal pain that would otherwise not occur. Some athletes feel that it is easier to run on a grass surface and will seek one out if they are trying to nurse a leg injury. In my experience, this only makes matters worse, since beneath the deceptive green covering, the underlying ground is often rutted and uneven, making each stride a hazard and increasing the stress on tendons and ligaments. If possible, then, do your training on the road or on a track with a good surface.

12. Facts and Fallacies

Over the years, I have developed the habit of holding informal chats before each exercise session to answer patients' questions and discuss the implications of recent studies and experiments on heart disease, fitness, and related subjects. The following topics are those most commonly covered in these sessions. I hope they will clarify a few of your problems and correct some of the half-truths, fallacies, and prejudices with which the exercising heart patient is surrounded.

Sexual Activity After Heart Attack

Half our postcoronary patients reported a reduction in sexual activity since their heart attacks. The main reason given was a fall-off in desire. A smaller number said that they were frightened of suffering another heart attack during intercourse, and a few actually reported adverse symptoms such as palpitations or angina pectoris during the sexual act.

The individual who becomes apathetic toward sex after the attack frequently shows high levels of depression and anxiety. The reluctance to seek full satisfaction in sexual relations is perfectly understandable under these circumstances. As confidence returns (and this often occurs with increasing physical fitness), the situation usually rights itself.

But what of the individual who is frightened of sexual intercourse because of its possible ill effects on the heart? Is there any justification for these fears? Should special precautions be observed during the sex act, and if so, what should they be? How long should one wait after the heart attack before resuming a normal sexual relationship?

The answers to these questions may have been provided by your cardiologist, but I find that many of the patients referred for rehabilitation have been given little guidance in this area. The reason is not hard to find. Minimal research has been carried out into the effects of coitus on the damaged heart, and medical literature contains little on the subject.

The sex act results in cardiovascular responses very similar to those induced by exercise. There is a rise in heart rate and blood pressure, as well as an increase in the rate of breathing. However, in terms of cardiac work, the cost of intercourse is modest, with increases in heart rate about the same as that observed in climbing a few flights of stairs or walking briskly around the block. As a matter of fact, much higher heart rates may occur during angry discussions at work! ECG monitoring of 14 subjects during the sexual act showed that a small number developed changes compatible with cardiac ischaemia (ST segment depression and ectopic beats), but these particular individuals experienced similar adverse signs during their usual occupational activities; in other words, coitus did not have a disproportionately higher stress effect.

The vast majority of postcoronary patients can safely indulge in marital sexual activity without fear of excessive cardiovascular strain. Here we refer to middle-aged individuals who have been married for a number of years. There are grounds for believing that intercourse with a younger or less familiar partner may lead to more profound physiological changes, with much higher increments of heart rate and blood pressure and so greater cardiac stress. Extra-marital intercourse may well provide these ingredients, and since it may also be accompanied by a bout of excessive food and alcohol intake, might well be dangerous. It is probably in these circumstances that the occasional coitus death occurs — a death dramatic enough to become more colorful in the retelling, and so needlessly frighten the more conservative members of society!

Are there precautions to be taken after a heart attack? Sufficient time should be allowed after the attack before indulging in intercourse. Wait three to four weeks after the attack, or until you can go for a brisk walk or climb two flights of stairs without difficulty. If you suffer from angina during coitus, then try taking glyceryl trinitrate before commencing the act. Symptoms such as angina or ectopic beats may be relieved by changing your position. Supporting your body weight on your arms amounts to isometric exercise and, as previously noted, will lead to a disproportionate increase in blood pressure and cardiac work load. The effect is enhanced if the duration of the act is prolonged. Therefore, if you are bothered by symptoms, try the side-by-side position or have your partner take the top position.

Depression Following Heart Attack

Our own studies, as well as the work of others, have shown that a significant number of heart attack survivors are extremely depressed as a result of their attacks. Actually, one-third of the group we analyzed demonstrated this finding. This state of affairs was evident only after careful evaluation; it was not obvious to the onlooker. As a matter of fact, neither the patients' spouses nor their physicians had even suspected it. When confronted with the evidence of the psychological assessment, the unhappy individual invariably admitted to melancholy.

The depressed heart patient lacks in confidence, shows less initiative at home and work, is reluctant to make important decisions, and constantly procrastinates, hoping that time will solve the problem. At home, more and more responsibility is left to the spouse. This change was so marked in one patient that his wife, before leaving for a holiday, wrote him a note in which she abjured him to pull himself together and revert to the strong-minded man she had married who had consistently called the shots for both of them. The trouble is that this is easier said than done. It takes time, a lot of patience and understanding, and sometimes the skill and advice of a professional.

There is little doubt that great benefit can be derived from an exercise rehabilitation program. Fitness improves the quality of life and brings with it enhanced self-confidence and improvement in morale. Our depressed patients have gained considerably from the exercise program. However, we have learned to take a slightly different approach with our depressed as opposed to our non-depressed patients. The latter have no sense of insecurity; psychological testing reveals that they have abundant self-confidence. Ambitious, driving, and overcompetitive, they deny adverse symptoms and are obsessive in their adherence to their exercise workouts. They are constantly matching their performances with those of others and setting themselves harder and harder goals. They are inclined to exceed their exercise prescription and have to be observed carefully in order to see that they do not do too much or ignore the indications for a reduction in training intensity.

The depressed patients are just the opposite, tending to be overly protective, frightened of exertion, doubtful of the program's value, pessimistic about their own chances of improvement, and inclined to do less than the prescription calls for. They allow any number of trivial excuses to deflect them from the exercise session, frequently complain of leg muscle stiffness, or vague discomfort in the chest, and constantly seem to be searching for an excuse to drop out. They need encouragement, reassurance, and a high degree of persuasion to see that they keep on exercising at a suitable level. They are helped by observing the success of other postcoronary joggers who are obviously doing so well. If they can just stay with the program long enough to start feeling the benefits of fitness, they are well on the road to recovery.

Do you recognize yourself as belonging to either of these two groups? If so, consider how your attitude affects your approach to exercise — and to your life in general.

Exercise-Related Deaths

Death during or shortly after a bout of exercise is a rare event. It is also a dramatic event and inevitably draws attention, particularly if the victim is famous, well-known, or a high-profile member of the community. Typical examples of the latter are Hank Gathers, the basketball star, and Jim Fixx, the author of the best-seller *The Book of Running*. By focusing attention on the advantages and disadvantages of exercise, the wide publicity given to these individuals' deaths served a valuable purpose. On the other hand, if it led people to believe that taking up exercise in order to become physically fit was a life-threatening procedure, it did a great disservice. Regular physical exercise is clearly an important part of a strategy for the prevention of coronary heart disease. Since one of the manifestations of that disease is sudden death, how can I reconcile this with the occasional accounts that this occurs while someone is exercising?

Let us put the topic in perspective. In the United States, one in every four people under the age of 50 years who dies of natural causes dies suddenly. The majority of these are due to diseases of the heart or blood vessels, and in those 30 years or older, practically all are due to coronary atherosclerosis. In most cases, the presence of coronary disease had already been diagnosed and the subject was aware of it, but in others there were no prior symptoms and the victim was apparently healthy. The latter cases are labeled medically as "sudden cardiac deaths" (SCDs).

SCD is so common these days that autopsy findings are of medical interest only if they reveal a non-cardiac cause. Furthermore, sudden death in patients with known coronary disease is so taken for granted that autopsy is rarely carried out. At times this can lead to false assumptions. An example is a 68-year-old TRC coronary patient who collapsed and died in the bathroom while getting ready to go out for his morning jog. It was presumed that he died as a result of his coronary disease. However, in life he had requested that autopsy be carried out if he died suddenly. The autopsy revealed that he had died from a very rare inflammatory disease of the heart muscle, sarcoidosis, which had nothing to do with his coronary atherosclerosis, and could have occurred at any time. Had it happened a short time later, while exercising, it would have been labeled an exercise death — and, incidentally, would have encouraged opponents of exercise to raise their voices in the usual chorus of "I told you so."

With SCD so common, the circumstances under which it happens are bound to be many and varied, but the nature of the activity that preceded the death may have had nothing to do with the event. In other words, we must not confuse association with cause. After all, if we can use the term "exercise death," why not a sleeping death, or a television-watching death, or a sitting-at-the-desk death, or a walking-the-dog death?

Because of the current worldwide interest in exercise for its health benefits, and the reports from time to time of exercise deaths, public health physicians, cardiology researchers, and statisticians have investigated the problem in some detail. The major difficulty has been to determine if the incidence of SCD is *relatively* more frequent during exercise than during sedentary activities. In absolute figures, there is no doubt that this is decidedly not the case.

In a study carried out in Rhode Island, with a population of approximately 1 million, there were only 81 exercise-related deaths over the period 1975 to 1982. Set against the overall SCD rate in the Rhode Island population as a whole, this is minuscule. Out of 7,629 joggers, there was only one exercise SCD per year.

One of the most informative studies was carried out by Dr. David Siscovik from the University of North Carolina, in association with the Department of Epidemiology, University of Washington. It looked at the incidence of SCD in King County, Washington, which has a population of 1¼ million.

Siscovik was able to show that those who habitually exercise to a moderate and high level are approximately half as likely to die suddenly from coronary disease, under any circumstances, as the sedentary or those with low-level physical activity patterns. However, if the moderate- or high-level exercisers do suffer a cardiac arrest, it is slightly more likely to occur during an exercise session. Does this mean that exercise is dangerous therapy? CABG surgery carries a 2% mortality risk, but no one would advocate that it be banned on that account. Vaccination for smallpox occasionally resulted in an extremely severe reaction, called vaccinia, which resembled smallpox and was occasionally fatal. If this had led to the withdrawal of vaccination as a routine procedure, we would never have been able to eliminate the smallpox virus from the entire planet. In other words, the advantages massively outweighed the disadvantages, and so it is with exercise.

A further observation from the King County Study, and one that has been reported frequently by other investigators, is that exercise SCD is more likely in those middle-aged, coronary-prone, sedentary individuals who exercise rarely, and when they do, at an unaccustomed and high level of intensity. Typically, these are the weekend athletes, who are inactive all winter, and then play a hard game of tennis on that first good weekend of summer.

People with normal hearts, for all practical purposes, do not suffer exercise SCD. Reports to the contrary are so rare, and so open to question, that they need not concern us here. In the under-30-year-olds, the causes are usually congenital malformation of the coronary vessels of the heart valves, myocarditis or inflammation of the heart muscle, or hypertrophic cardiomyopathy, a disease that enlarges the muscle fibers of the heart and thickens its walls (and which, incidentally, caused the death of Hank Gathers).

In the over-30-year-olds, rare as exercise SCD is, we know that it is almost always associated with the presence of coronary heart disease, recognized or otherwise. The evidence from cardiac exercise programs such as mine, however, shows quite clearly that coronary patients can and do exercise regularly with minimal risk. The incidence of exercise-associated deaths is appreciably lower than that in the population in general. However, caution is imperative, and all of these patients have the advantage of undergoing an exercise test, with electrocardiographic monitoring during exercise sessions when indicated, and a medically prescribed, carefully supervised regime. They are taught to recognize and report dangerous symptoms and have a set of rules to follow that reduce their risk of exercise SCD. For those not on such a program, however, the points covered in Chapter 9 should be carefully considered.

If you are a middle-aged casual exerciser, beginner or otherwise, you should not engage in vigorous games such as squash, or indeed any competitive sport, unless you are fit enough to do so. You can check your fitness level by having a formal fitness test at your local "Y," local health club, or better still, in your physician's office. If this is not possible, then you can carry out the fitness step test outlined in this book, or refer to the cardiovascular fitness tables in the appendices.

The problems of exercising in the heat have been discussed elsewhere but one cannot overemphasize the dangers. Deaths during exercise in high temperatures have been ascribed to heart attacks, and yet on more than one occasion autopsies have failed to reveal any evidence of coronary atherosclerosis. It is not unreasonable to assume that such deaths have been due to dehydration, alteration in blood electrolytes, and maybe even coronary spasm. No one is immune to all the consequences of dehydration, but middle-aged individuals with latent coronary artery disease are more susceptible.

Another important factor to take into consideration is that of personality. The driving, ambitious individual, once introduced to an exercise program, is usually overeager to excel. If you are one of these, then you will be well-advised to control your tendency toward aggression and competitiveness; it is easy for you to become compulsive and, when business pressures mount, try to complete your workout in a shorter and shorter time. Even worse, you may deny cardiac symptoms in order to keep up your exercise program and still handle heavy business and social commitments. The inherent danger in this attitude is that it always causes a delay before symptoms are brought to the attention of the physician. I suspect that the ill-fated Jim Fixx fell into this category. *Warning signs such as excessive fatigue, tiredness, and especially anginal-type chest pain on exercise should be taken very seriously. They are indications that the training must be immediately suspended, pending a detailed re-examination of your cardiovascular status.*

I have evolved five exercise rules that apply particularly to these highly competitive, "deadline" personalities:

- Train regularly without excessive peaks of activity.
- Avoid intensive competition.
- Adhere to the prescribed limits.
- Reduce the exercise load when physical symptoms, mental tension, or physical tension develops.

- Report all "cardiac-type" symptoms such as exercise-related chest pain, arm pain, excessive palpitations, dizziness, "blackouts," or undue breathlessness — even if they appear for the first time after years of steady symptom-free training.

To sum up, exercise-induced deaths are very rare, but they do occur and are more likely in the non-conditioned coronary-prone individual, with and without previous evidence of coronary heart disease. Nevertheless, the fact that the recent worldwide explosion in all forms of exercise has not been accompanied by an immediate and proportionate increase in exercise SCD attests in the most dramatic and convincing way possible to the inherent safety of sensible moderate physical training programs.

Participation in Other Sporting Activities

When can I play tennis? What about golf? Is badminton okay? How about swimming? These and other similar questions are asked constantly by postcoronary patients who are on the exercise program. We try to answer each one individually, taking into account the patient's state of training, age, severity of heart attack, and presence or absence of symptoms. If you are working out in accordance with the training tables in this book, then you can use your achievement of the various levels as a rough guide to your ability to participate safely in a number of recreational physical activities (see Appendix E).

Although some of these recreational physical activities may be more enjoyable than jogging, they are harder to quantify in terms of energy expenditure and cardiac work. If you are good at a game, then you will perform it with greater skill, or to put it physiologically, with a higher degree of mechanical efficiency. Thus your oxygen intake will be lower throughout the game than if you were a less proficient player. A poor swimmer will expend more effort thrashing across the pool than his or her accomplished counterpart in an apparently lazy workout covering many lengths. The squash player with 20 years' experience will finish a game hardly perspiring, while his or her sweating novice opponent may have just had the match of his life.

Other variables in recreational sports include difficulty in pacing oneself, the effect of emotion and excitement, as well as extraneous factors peculiar to the game itself — as for example, the isometric component involved in gripping the golf club or the ski-tow bar, or the late nights (and possibly the hip-flask conviviality) associated with club curling.

Air Travel

Nowadays, whether for business or vacation, most of us have to fly at some time or another. Can flying pose any special threat for the individual with coronary artery disease? Generally speaking, the answer is no. However, certain considerations have to be taken into account.

Jet planes usually cruise at altitudes of between 30,000 and 40,000 feet (9,144 to 12,192 meters). At these heights, the atmosphere is so rarefied that, were it not for the pressurized cabin, passengers and crew would rapidly expire due to lack of oxygen. Pressurization ensures that the cabin altitude remains at between 5,000 and 7,000 feet (1,524 to 2,134 meters). While it is possible to pressurize the cabin to sea level when flying at heights in excess of 25,000 feet (7,620 meters), it is not economical to do so; and, indeed, for most travelers it is not necessary. In effect, the majority of trips are made at cabin altitudes between that equivalent to Denver, Colorado (5,000 feet or 1,524 meters), and slightly less than Mexico City (7,523 feet or 2,293 meters). This is not a serious problem, since our blood's ability to absorb and transport oxygen through the circulatory system isn't materially hindered until we are exposed to altitudes of 10,000 feet (3,048 meters) and above.

However, individuals with chest disease, such as chronic bronchitis or emphysema, may have difficulty getting sufficient oxygen at lower atmospheric pressures than 10,000 feet (3,048 meters). Obviously, any chest patient who is breathless at rest, or on minimal exertion, will fly only after very careful medical assessment. As for those with coronary artery disease, the ability to climb two flights of stairs easily or walk 100 yards (91 meters) briskly without breathlessness should ensure a problem-free flight.

How long after a heart attack should one wait before flying? Published reports indicate that fewer problems occur in those whose heart attack has happened two to six months before the flight, than in those who fly less than eight weeks after their attack. Those in whom the attack was accompanied by complications, or in whom there was a history of more than one previous attack, also have a higher occurrence of in-flight problems. It would seem wise, then, to defer flying for at least two months. However, British Airways recommends that if the journey is essential, an uncomplicated case can fly as early as two weeks postinfarction.

Actually, in my experience, patients have suffered more episodes of angina on the ground than in the air, as a result of the strain and frustrations of crowded airports, flight delays, customs and immigration inspections, and lengthy waits at baggage conveyors.

Apart from the matter of cabin altitude, there are other aspects of air travel that are probably more important. Alcohol and cigarette smoke intensify the ill effects of low blood oxygen, and so are best avoided, or at least reduced, during long flights. Since the atmosphere in the cabin is dry and rarefied, dehydration can be a problem. Remember, then, to drink plenty of non-alcoholic fluid. Another point to note is that gas expands at altitude. That includes the gas in your stomach. Therefore, on a long flight wear loose clothing, and don't consume too many carbonated drinks, or you'll bloat up like a balloon. Take a walk up and down the cabin every half hour or so to keep the circulation flowing and to avoid blood "pooling" in the lower limbs. If this is not possible, straighten your knees and ankles and clench the thigh and calf muscles from time to time. Finally, and most importantly, always carry three days' supply of your medication on your person or in your cabin luggage. If you pack it in checked luggage, you will sooner or later face the problem of lost bags and, at best, the inconvenience of having to find a local physician to prescribe replacements.

DIETARY SUPPLEMENTS

This is indeed a tangled web, spun by researchers, evangelists, and ignoramuses alike. Nevertheless, the subject warrants consideration and so, without fear or favor or more ado, here are some thoughts for your consideration.

Vitamin C

This substance is essential in the manufacture of collagen, the base substance that acts as a cement for much of the tissue and organs of our bodies. It occurs naturally in citrus fruit such as lemons and limes. It was not until 1932 that the specific protective agent in the lime was isolated in the form of Vitamin C; two years later, it was first synthesized.

Recently, there has been renewed interest in Vitamin C for a number of reasons. The world-famous scientist and Nobel Prize winner Dr. Linus Pauling has advocated the therapeutic use of large doses of Vitamin C to help the body's defense mechanisms against infection. Once again, this subject is obscured by controversy. Time and time again, you will come across the arguments for and against the use of so-called megavitamin therapy. Orthodox medical teaching has established minimal daily requirements for all of the known vitamins. It has also identified a number of clear-cut conditions that result if these minimal daily requirements are not met. Scurvy, beri-beri (lack of Vitamin B), rickets (Vitamin D), night blindness (Vitamin A), are all examples of gross deficiency in vitamins. The megavitamin advocates, however, maintain that disease entities exist that are less dramatic and obvious in appearance and are caused by a chronic partial shortage of dietary vitamins. They aim to correct these conditions by supplementing the diet with large doses of the vitamin in question.

Their arguments are still tenuous, and valid scientific data to prove their point are still lacking. Nevertheless, to be fair, while large numbers of ill-trained enthusiasts and outright cranks are advocating all sorts of vitamin therapy for a host of conditions, both real and imagined, an increasing number of reputable physicians and scientists are devoting their attention to a careful study of the topic. The opinion of an individual such as Dr. Linus Pauling cannot be ignored.

To return to Vitamin C. It is not too surprising to find that some researchers have claimed coronary artery disease to be a Vitamin C deficiency state. Their argument is that adequate quantities of this substance in the body will protect against atherosclerosis. Again, there is no proof that this is so. However, there are certain facts about Vitamin C that are worthy of note. High levels of physical stress will result in a depletion of the body's stores of Vitamin C. Thus, an exhausting long-distance run, or two or three nights without sleep, will deplete our Vitamin C reserves. Our bodies cannot manufacture Vitamin C; we must obtain it from the environment, either in natural or synthetic form. Consequently, it is reasonable to argue that individuals who are under high physical stress will require increased doses of the vitamin. Another point to bear in mind is that smoking and alcohol both destroy Vitamin C.

With these facts in mind, it does seem reasonable to take Vitamin C as a supplement when you are under physical stress. In our context, this would include heavy training. The person who is jogging three or more miles (five kilometers or more) five days a week would be included in that category. I recommend to my patients who are running five to six miles (eight to ten kilometers), five times a week, that they take 500 mg daily. If they are running longer distances, then I recommend higher dosages.

What about the cost and the safety factors? Of all the vitamins, surely Vitamin C must be the cheapest, so that does not constitute a problem. On the matter of safety, there are one or two provisos. The body can store only so much ascorbic acid in the tissues, and any excess is excreted in the urine. This tends to make the urine acid, and some authorities have stated that this could lead to the formation of certain types of kidney stones. While this is a remote hazard, it can be reduced by maintaining an adequate fluid intake. Further, stone formation seems to me to be likely only when the intake of the vitamin is truly massive.

The influence of high dosage is probably also a factor in a more cogent objection, namely that the body becomes accustomed to high Vitamin C levels, and if the high dosage is suddenly withdrawn, then a mild type of scurvy may occur. Again, this seems unlikely with dosages in the order of half a gram to a gram.

Vitamin E
Few subjects arouse more passion in medical circles than that dealing with the possible therapeutic value of this substance. The proponents of Vitamin E therapy angrily denounce their antagonists as being short-sighted and accuse them of deliberately ignoring the evidence of innumerable case histories in which large doses of Vitamin E

have been of value in heart disease, leg ulcers, skin infections, and a whole host of other conditions. The opposition, however (and that probably includes the bulk of the medical profession), counters with the argument that there is a paucity of controlled clinical trials demonstrating that Vitamin E therapy is of any value, that deficiency states occur only rarely, and that Vitamin E is obtained in sufficient quantities from a normal diet without further supplementation. The battle has raged since 1922 when the substance, known as tocopherol, was discovered. Present in large amounts in wheat germ and green leaves, its absence from the diet of laboratory rats was shown to cause sterility and a peculiar condition in which the muscles become swollen and weak.

The current rationale for the use of Vitamin E in the treatment of atherosclerosis is based on the theory that the present epidemiology of coronary artery disease is largely due to a deficiency in this vitamin, resulting from our modern diet. The milling and purification of flour and other foodstuffs has led to the elimination of Vitamin E, it is argued, so that we now have a need to supplement this factor artificially. Among its reputedly beneficial effects are a reduction in the tendency for blood to clot, a dilation of peripheral blood vessels, and a reduction in the oxygen requirements of the tissue cells. Unfortunately, none of these properties has been consistently demonstrated by laboratory trials.

When faced with the question of whether it is advisable to take a substance that has not as yet received the universal blessing of the medical profession, I am forced to fall back on two questions: Is it safe? And, is it expensive? Certainly, no toxic effects from the use of large doses of Vitamin E have ever been recorded in human beings. I am told by a good physician friend of mine who prescribes Vitamin E for many conditions, that it should be used with caution in patients with high blood pressure, at least in the initial stages of treatment; and that it is not indicated in patients with certain types of valvular disease of the heart.

High intake of Vitamin E has been linked to a drop in the body's Vitamin K content. Vitamin K helps blood to clot, and so it is just conceivable that tocopherol, in destroying Vitamin K, may reduce the likelihood of thrombosis occurring within the coronary arteries. A more immediate implication of this finding, however, is that patients who have been placed on anticoagulant medication ("blood thinner") after their heart attacks might well be cautious about taking non-prescribed megadoses of Vitamin E for fear that the cumulative effect will result in excessive bleeding.

With the above proviso, I think we can conclude that Vitamin E is safe; but it is not cheap. However, if you have to cut down your smoking in order to afford a year's supply of Vitamin E capsules, then it is money well spent.

Lecithin

Many health food advocates have promoted the use of lecithin for the prevention and treatment of coronary heart disease. Chemically, lecithin is similar to a triglyceride (glycerol combined with three fatty acids), except that it also includes two additional substances, phosphoric acid and choline. Lecithin is found in brain and nervous tissue and in egg yolk, and its purpose is to help in the transfer of fat around the body. In industry, lecithin is used widely as an emulsifying agent; by lowering surface tension, it allows two liquids that are initially soluble to mix, e.g., the butter fat and water in milk. The lecithin used in industry is derived from soy bean oil, and therefore the fatty acid in its molecule is polyunsaturated. The rationale for taking lecithin is that it will emulsify the fat in the intestine and in the blood and thus prevent it from building up to form atherosclerotic deposits on the walls of the arteries. A simple understanding of body chemistry quickly dispels this theory.

The lecithin you eat is digested by the stomach acids and enzymes and so broken down into its four components, glycerol, fatty acids, phosphoric acid, and choline. These substances are then transported to the liver where they are reassembled to make the body's own lecithin. Thus, it cannot "emulsify" fat as it does in a test tube or in a frying pan. The only benefit, if any, of taking soy bean lecithin lies in the fact that you are increasing your intake of polyunsaturated fatty acids. On the other hand, if you eat lecithin of animal origin, then you are doing more harm than good since you are increasing your intake of saturated fatty acids. So why pay health food prices for lecithin tablets, granules, or some other form, when you might as well get your polyunsaturated fatty acids from soy bean or any other vegetable oil?

CHELATION THERAPY

This controversial method of treating coronary atherosclerosis involves the use of a substance called EDTA, which was formerly used for the treatment of metal poisoning. It is a chelating agent, which means that when it is injected into the bloodstream, it combines with the metal and facilitates its elimination from the body. When used in the treatment of coronary disease, it is transfused into an arm vein with the intention that it will combine with and remove the calcium in the atherosclerotic deposits. In this way the deposit, or plaque, will shrink and the coronary narrowings improve. The treatment lasts for about 30 minutes and the number of sessions depends on the progress being made, but could be as many as 30 or more. This method, although carried out by some doctors, has not met with the approval of any cardiac society or university medical department, national or international. It is not covered by the Canadian health insurance system, nor by any of the major insurance companies in the United States, including Medicare.

Why the controversy? There is no doubt that chelation therapy is an attractive alternative for some patients faced with coronary artery bypass surgery. Yet there is little or no scientific evidence that chelation can actually remove calcium from atherosclerotic deposits. Even if by some remote possibility it could, that still would not improve the situation. You will remember from our earlier discussions that these deposits consist largely of fatty debris, smooth muscle cells, fibrous tissue, and cell remnants. Calcium is a late addition to the process, and then occurs only in small amounts.

This is not to say that patients who attend chelation clinics cannot improve. If they also go on a low-fat diet, start an exercise program, stop smoking, and, if necessary, have their hypertension and diabetes treated, then obviously, chelation therapy or not, they can expect a benefit. The mere fact that they often attend the clinic for a lengthy period ensures their continued contact with the nurse and physician, thus reinforcing their motivation to maintain a healthy lifestyle.

On the other hand, I end this topic on a note of caution. Patients who have critical atherosclerotic lesions of their coronary arteries, who are candidates for bypass surgery or angioplasty, and who choose to undergo a course of chelation therapy instead, are delaying effective proven therapy that could conceivably save their life.

13. Family Matters

This chapter is for husbands, wives, and other relatives of heart patients, and in some ways it is probably one of the most important in the entire book. Why so? Because a change in lifestyle in a partnership means a change for both parties. I will go further. Only with the complete cooperation and understanding of the spouse can the heart attack patient hope to adhere to this or any other cardiac rehabilitation program.

In the Hospital

The problems start immediately with the diagnosis of the heart attack. Nearly half the spouses we interviewed reported being numbed, or in a state of shock on hearing the news. Like the victims, they echo the phrase, "This can't be happening." This sense of unreality is quickly shattered, however, by the day-to-day problems that arise. Most difficult perhaps are the visits to the hospital, which have to be fitted in between the usual daily duties, whether holding down a job, looking after the kids, or, more commonly these days, both.

How should you behave during these hospital visits? Above all, your attitude should express confident anticipation of an excellent recovery. In the vast majority of cases, that will be the outcome. Only if the doctors and nurses caution against any optimism should you adopt a sober, realistic approach. Even then, remember that doctors, like weather forecasters, are never right 100% of the time. So feel free to be optimistic and to discuss plans for what you both will do after leaving the hospital. Something good to look forward to is probably the best of all medicines. In the early days in hospital, however, and immediately after coming out of critical care, fatigue is a common symptom. Don't overstay your welcome.

At Home

For the first few weeks after discharge, the patient may be overly dependent and even childlike in attitude. Don't encourage this dependency or be too fearful. As one wife said, "I am scared stiff that I will lose my temper, raise my voice, criticize or do anything that will make him ill again."

A feature of the Toronto program is an evening with the spouses of newly referred patients. It provides an occasion to meet with the staff, and allows me an opportunity to explain the nature of heart disease, its possible causes, and the role that exercise and risk reduction play in prevention. After the talk, the questions start. With audiences of about one hundred assembled, you can imagine that the queries are many and varied. Here are some of the questions most often asked by the concerned partner.

How Can I Overcome Despondency?

It is now accepted that rehabilitation should start as soon as the patient gets out of the coronary care unit and returns to the general ward. For the moment, the patient is glad just to be alive, but as the days pass, that feeling of relief is replaced by one of despondency. The mind is plagued by doubts and uncertainties, all revolving around the ability to do all the things that were part and parcel of everyday life before the attack. As one patient said to me, "I desperately wanted to get out of the hospital, and yet I was scared to go home. Things I had always taken for granted now became a first. The first time you walk up the stairs, or mow the grass, or clean out the basement, or go back to work, it's the same feeling — will you make it? It's as if you're trying to pick up the pieces of your life again, and never being sure if they'll fit together properly this time."

A good postcoronary rehabilitation program helps to overcome much of this fear. No program, however, can help as much as a well-informed spouse. Take a positive approach right from hospital discharge. Don't avoid discussing the future. The majority of heart attack patients return to their previous lives. If your spouse's is the exceptional case, it still does no harm to discuss alternatives. To make small talk and steer away from a topic as important as future work plans is a great mistake; to the depressed patient, it can only mean one thing — there is no future to discuss.

Avoid being over-solicitous. Exercise sensible precautions, but don't fuss. No doubt certain physical activities are slightly more risky, but then driving an automobile isn't exactly 100% safe these days, and no one can live life completely immune from risk. Besides, until recently, the tendency has been to exaggerate the dangers of physical effort for heart attack patients. We now know that many of the things that they want to do are perfectly safe. Your doctor, or the rehabilitation team, should be able to advise you if there are any important physical restrictions.

In the first few months after the attack, there is often a reluctance to make decisions. This is perfectly natural and is just another manifestation of the depressed mood.

Eventually, the situation rights itself. Be patient, and whatever you do, don't get into the habit of making all the decisions in the home. If you do, you may well find yourself stuck with the role of decision maker permanently. Every so often, give your partner the opportunity to regain the initiative.

How Should I React to Symptoms?

Symptom-claiming is not unusual in the early days following the attack. It is an expression of insecurity and represents a need for reassurance. This phase may last a matter of months only, but it can be a real trial for the spouse who never becomes quite accustomed to a succession of frightening complaints of chest pain, numbness in hands, dizziness, and so on. It is difficult not to push the panic button and call the physician on every occasion.

There are, however, some guidelines for action. Severe chest pain (or pain similar to that which accompanied the first attack) that lasts for more than 20 minutes, is not relieved by taking nitroglycerine, lying down or resting, and is accompanied by sweating, pallor, nausea, or vomiting indicates the need for speedy medical assistance. If you can't get the physician, arrange immediate transportation to the emergency department.

There are other indications of impending trouble that, although less dramatic than chest pain, should nevertheless be heeded. Foremost among these is excessive fatigue. Tiredness that is not relieved by a good night's rest should be considered suspect in the recent postcoronary patient, and a search should be made for the cause. A heavy work load or an overcrowded social itinerary is usually the culprit, and steps should be taken immediately to adopt a more sensible and relaxed routine. Frequently, the spouse is the first to recognize the onset of the cantankerous, irritable manner that was so typical of the first attack. Both fatigue and irritability may be the result of a return to the old lifestyle, with its worries, real or imagined, heavy work schedule, and absence of physical activity and recreation — in short, a repetition of the very set of circumstances that probably triggered the initial acute attack.

Is it not better to be sure than sorry? Within reason, yes. However, a patient cannot keep running in and out of the doctor's office or the hospital emergency department. He or she must learn to exercise judgment and maturity in assessing the significance of various symptoms. Getting into the habit of requiring an electrocardiogram for every ache or pain is the path to cardiac neurosis — in my experience, one of the most difficult of all conditions to cure. If this preoccupation with symptoms that consistently prove to be groundless persists beyond a six-month period or so, and shows no signs of responding to simple reassurance on your part, then it should be mentioned to the family physician or the cardiologist. Psychological treatment may be indicated to relieve the condition before the pattern becomes set.

What About Sexual Activity?

Many postcoronary patients, both male and female, quickly regain their interest in sex after the acute stage of the attack is over and they have returned home to their routine daily activities. The chances are that their level of interest will be the same as previously. This subject is dealt with on pages 291–293, but spouses may have concerns of their own. Most such concerns are largely groundless. Unless the heart has been extensively damaged, there is no more danger after the heart attack than there was before it. So don't enter the situation in obvious fear and trepidation. Nothing is more destined to put your partner off and increase feelings of depression, insecurity, and worthlessness.

There are certain medications that, in some patients, may reduce sexual urge. The individual variations are wide, and it is frequently very difficult to distinguish between a true chemical side effect and a host of other less tangible causes. However, there have been reports of reduction in libido following the taking of various drugs used to lower blood pressure, certain beta-blockers, as well as some cholesterol-lowering agents, tranquilizers, and antidepressants. If one of these medications is suspected in reducing sexual desire, the matter should be discussed with the prescribing physician. On no account allow your spouse to stop a medication on the grounds of suspicion. It is often relatively easy for the physician to substitute another substance that is equally effective but does not carry the same side effects. While we are on the subject, incidentally, let me remind you that the two most common drugs that have been shown to reduce sexual appetite are non-prescription — alcohol and cigarettes!

How Can I Prevent Another Attack?

Recognition of dangerous symptoms is one thing; preventing them from appearing is a far more worthwhile goal. What positive steps should you take to help your partner keep from having a further attack? It can be expressed in a phrase: "Give all assistance in efforts to change lifestyle." The previous way of life contained the seeds of the attack. You now have a chance to help alter the situation. This means a prudent diet low in cholesterol and animal fats, a physical-fitness program, a total veto on cigarette smoking (this applies to you, also), and moderation in both work and play.

You will need to accommodate this new partner. The more accommodation needed, the more you can console yourself with the thought that the rehabilitation is proceeding successfully. You may have to arrange mealtimes to fit in with the exercise sessions. If you can't walk together, then take the trouble to acquaint yourself with the time the workout should take, and then plan accordingly.

Another side effect of increasing fitness is the desire to take up new and sometimes more strenuous leisure activities, such as camping, sailboating, backpacking, and cross-country skiing. Often allied with this is an increased interest in the simpler pleasures; walking in the rain, reading a good novel, taking a fall outing on foot to catch the colors.

It's not always easy to change, even for a good reason. I still recall with crystal clarity the bemused tone with which one of my earliest "successes" described his wife's reaction to his newly awakened yearnings. "You know what she said, Doc?" he intoned sadly. "'I wish you hadn't changed. We were so happy when you were the way you used to be.'" The way he "used to be" had set the stage for his heart attack!

Contrast this with the sentiments of another couple who told me that the heart attack, initially a devastating event, ultimately turned out to have a beneficial effect. It brought them closer together, gave them a new set of values based on health rather than wealth, and led them to adopt a far more fulfilling lifestyle. If this book helps you to achieve a similar result, it will have served its purpose well.

APPENDIX A: NOMOGRAMS

NOMOGRAM A
To Be Used for Calculating Your Progressing Heart Rate

Age	Progressing Heart Rate (beats per minute)	Resting Heart Rate (beats per minute)
25	150	95
30	145	90
35	140	85
40	135	80
45	130	75
50	125	72
55	120	
60	115	
65		

For those who have completed a stress test without adverse symptoms or who are free from heart disease.

A line joining your resting heart rate and your age will intersect the center column at your progressing heart rate. Resting heart rates below 72 beats per minute should be charted at 72.

To obtain your heart rate (pulse rate) and resting heart rate, see instructions on pages 188–189 and 243–245.

NOMOGRAM B

To Be Used for Calculating Your Training Heart Rate and Your Progressing Heart Rate

Maximum Heart Rate (Symptom Limited)
(beats per minute)

TRAINING HEART RATE
(beats per minute)

PROGRESSING HEART RATE
(beats per minute)

RESTING HEART RATE
(beats per minute)

For those who have not been able to complete a stress test because of the development of adverse symptoms or who have anginal pain, palpitations or breathlessness, etc.

A line joining your resting heart rate and the heart rate at which your symptoms appear, your maximum heart rate (symptom limited), will intersect the center columns at your training heart rate and progressing heart rate. Resting heart rates above 72 beats per minute should be charted at 72.

If the difference between your resting heart rate and your maximum heart rate (symptom limited) is less than 40 beats per minute, you should not attempt the training program in this book, except under medical supervision.

To obtain your heart rate (pulse rate) and resting heart rate, see instructions on pages 188–189 and 243–245.

Appendix A (cont'd.)

NOMOGRAM C
Nomogram for Prediction of Maximum Oxygen Intake in Men Aged 25 and 35 Years

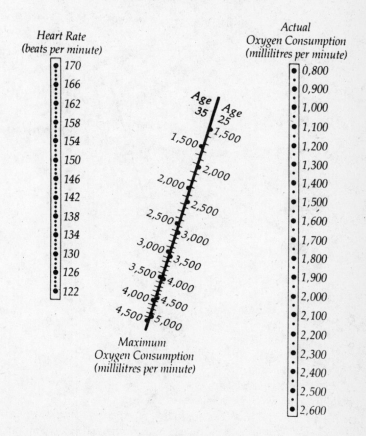

A line joining your heart rate and actual oxygen intake will intersect the center line at your maximum oxygen intake.

Appendix A (cont'd.)

NOMOGRAM D
Nomogram for Prediction of Maximum Oxygen Intake in Women Aged 25 and 35 Years

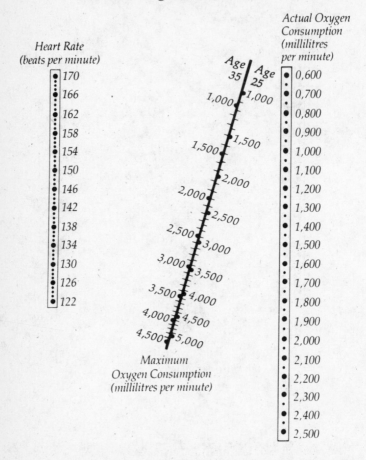

Heart Rate
(beats per minute)

Age 35   Age 25

Actual Oxygen
Consumption
(millilitres
per minute)

Maximum
Oxygen Consumption
(millilitres per minute)

A line joining your heart rate and actual oxygen intake will intersect the center line at your maximum oxygen intake.

Appendix A (cont'd.)

NOMOGRAM E
Nomogram for Prediction of Maximum Oxygen Intake in Men Aged 45 and 55 Years

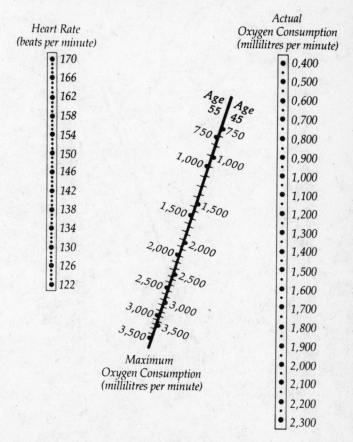

A line joining your heart rate and actual oxygen intake will intersect the center line at your maximum oxygen intake.

Appendix A (cont'd.)

NOMOGRAM F
Nomogram for Prediction of Maximum Oxygen Intake in Women Aged 45 and 55 Years

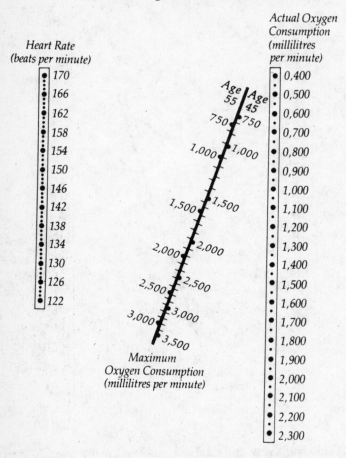

Maximum
Oxygen Consumption
(millilitres per minute)

A line joining your heart rate and actual oxygen intake will intersect the center line at your maximum oxygen intake.

APPENDIX B: TRAINING TABLES

To be used for determining your exercise prescription, *but* only after careful reading of the text.

If your predicted maximum oxygen consumption (VO_2 max) is below 16 milliliters per kilogram per minute, or if you do not actually know what it is, begin at the Preliminary Phase, Level 1. If your maximum oxygen consumption is more than 16 milliliters per kilogram per minute, begin at the appropriate level in Phase 1 (see pages 238–242).

Ideally, in all phases you should plan to exercise 5 times weekly.

Preliminary Phase
Levels to be taken in sequence.
Level 1   For 2 weeks walk 1 mile (1.6 km) in 30 minutes
Level 2   For 2 weeks walk 1½ miles (2.4 km) in 42 minutes
Level 3   For 2 weeks walk 2 miles (3.2 km) in 50 minutes
Level 4   For 2 weeks walk 2½ miles (4.0 km) in
            57½ minutes
When you have completed the Preliminary Phase, progress to Phase 1, Level 1.

Phase 1

For instructions on progressing through the levels of Phase 1, see page 245.

If you begin your exercise program at one of the levels in Phase 1 (see page 238), do not attempt at first the full prescription for your starting level. Instead, start with one-third the starting prescription (e.g., at Level 1, walk 1 mile [1.6 km] in 20 minutes if you are under age 45). After two weeks, progress to two-thirds the starting prescription (e.g., 2 miles [3.2 km] in 40 minutes, if under age 45 and

Appendix B (cont'd.)

at Level 1) for a further two weeks. Then, provided there are no adverse symptoms, proceed to the full three miles (4.8 km) in the time prescribed for your starting level.

Phase 1

Level	Predicted maximum oxygen consumption (milliliters per kilogram per minute)	Distance (miles)	Time (minutes)	
			Under age 45	Over age 45
1	16.1 to 17.5 mL/kg/min	3	60	63
2	17.6 to 18.4 mL/kg/min	3	57	60
3	18.5 to 21.3 mL/kg/min	3	54	57
4	21.4 to 22.7 mL/kg/min	3	51	54
5	22.8 to 25.6 mL/kg/min	3	48	51
6	25.7 to 28.5 mL/kg/min	3	45	48
7	28.6 + mL/kg/min	3	42	45

The transition stage from walking to jogging can be a little complicated, and so patients attending the Centre are given the following instructions:

Please note that in the following exercise prescriptions, walking is done at a 15-minutes-per-mile/9:15-minutes-per-kilometer pace, and jogging at 12-minutes-per-mile/7:30-minutes-per-kilometer pace. All speeds for the mile/1.6 kilometer and 3-mile/4.8-kilometer distances are rounded off to the nearest minute or quarter-minute. It is essential to keep as closely as possible to the 15-minutes-per-mile/9:15-minutes-per-kilometer pace for walking, and the 12-minutes-per-mile/7:30-minutes-per-kilometer pace for jogging. The 13½-minutes-per-mile/8:30-minutes-per-kilometer pace is repeated in the tables so as to effect a smoother transition from half-lap (100-meter/110-yard) jogs to whole-lap (200-meter/220-yard) jogs.

Appendix B (cont'd.)

1) 14½-minute-mile/9-minute-kilometer (43½ minutes for 3 miles/4.8 kilometers). Alternate 3½ laps walking with a half-lap jogging for a total of 24 laps to give 3 miles/ 4.8 kilometers.

2) 14-minute-mile/8:45-minute-kilometer (42 minutes for 3 miles/4.8 kilometers). Alternate 1½ laps walking with a half-lap jogging for a total of 24 laps to give 3 miles/ 4.8 kilometers.

3a) 13½-minute-mile/8:30-minute-kilometer (40½ minutes for 3 miles/4.8 kilometers). Alternate half-lap walk with half-lap jog for a total of 24 laps to give 3 miles/4.8 kilometers.

3b) 13½-minute-mile/8:30-minute-kilometer (40½ minutes for 3 miles/4.8 kilometers). Alternate one lap walk with one lap jog for a total of 24 laps to give 3 miles/4.8 kilometers.

4) 13-minute-mile/8-minute-kilometer (39 minutes for 3 miles/4.8 kilometers). Alternate half-lap walk with 1½ laps jogging for a total of 24 laps to give 3 miles/4.8 kilometers.

5) 12-minute-mile/7:30-minute-kilometer (36 minutes for 3 miles/4.8 kilometers). Jog the entire distance.

If you don't attend the Centre's program, but have access to a 200- or 400-meter/220- or 440-yard track, then you should adhere to the above instructions. However, if you are using the sidewalk or park as your training course, you will have to use a slightly different approach. Your first most important task is to familiarize yourself with the 15 minutes-per-mile (9:15-minutes-per-kilometer) walking pace and then with the 12-minutes-per-mile (7:30-minutes-per-kilometer) jogging pace. The latter is equivalent to jogging 100 meters/110 yards in 45 seconds. Once you have

Appendix B (cont'd.)

mastered this, then the five stages outlined above can be expressed as follows:

1) 14½-minute-mile/9-minute-kilometer (43½ minutes for 3 miles/4.8 kilometers). Alternate 6½ minutes walk (700 meters/770 yards at a 15-minute-mile/9:15-minute-kilometer pace) with a 45-second jog (100 meters/110 yards at a 12-minute-mile/7:30-minute-kilometer pace) for a total of 24 laps to give 3 miles/4.8 kilometers.

2) 14-minute-mile/8:45-minute-kilometer (42 minutes for 3 miles/4.8 kilometers). Alternate 2:45 walk (300 meters/ 330 yards), with 45-second jog (100 meters/110 yards) for a total of 24 laps to give 3 miles/4.8 kilometers.

3a) 13½-minute-mile/8:30-minute-kilometer (40½ minutes for 3 miles/4.8 kilometers). Alternate a 56-second walk (100 meters/110 yards) with a 45-second jog (100 meters/ 110 yards) for a total of 24 laps to give 3 miles.

3b) 13½-minute-mile/8:30-minute-kilometer (40½ minutes for 3 miles/4.8 kilometers). Alternate 1:53 walk (200 meters/220 yards), with a 90-second jog (200 meters/ 220 yards) for a total of 24 laps to give 3 miles/4.8 kilometers.

Appendix B (cont'd.)

Phase 2

For instructions on progressing through the levels of Phase 2, see pages 245–246.

Level							
					Over Age 45		
		Distance	Time	Approx. Pace (mins./ mile)	Distance	Time	Approx. Pace (mins./ mile)
	(miles)	(meters)*	(minutes)		(miles)	(minutes)	
1	3	4828	43½	14½	3	43½	14½
2	3	4828	42	14	3	42	14
3	3	4828	40½	13½(a)	3	40½	13½(a)
4	3	4828	40½	13½(b)	3	40½	13½(b)
5	3	4828	39	13	3	39	13
6	3	4828	36	12	3	36	12
7	3¼	5230	39	12	3¼	39	12
8	3½	5633	42	12	3½	42	12
9	3¾	6035	45	12	3¾	45	12
10	4	6437	48	12	4	48	12
11	4	6437	46	11½			
12	4	6437	44	11			
13	4	6437	42	10½	*Metric equivalents are		
14	4	6437	40	10	approximate.		

(column headers: Under Age 45 spans Distance (miles), Distance (meters), Time (minutes), Approx. Pace (mins./mile))*

After Phase 2, Level 11, you may progress to Phase 3.

Phase 3

For more instructions on progressing through the levels of Phase 3, see page 239.

Level			Under Age 45	Over Age 45
		Distance	Time	Time
	(miles)	(meters)	(minutes)	(minutes)
1	4¼	6800	42½	51
2	4½	7200	45	54
3	4¾	7600	47½	57
4	5	8000	50	60
5	5½	8800	55	66
6	6	9600	60	72

APPENDIX C: HEAT SAFETY INDEX

Heat Safety Index

APPENDIX D: WIND CHILL FACTORS

Wind Speed mph (km/h)*	Temperature °F (°C)*				
Calm	40(5)	35(2)	30(−1)	25(−4)	20(−7)
5(8)	35	30	25	20	15
10(16)	30	20	15	10	5
15(24)	25	15	10	0	−5
20(32)	20	10	5	0	−10
25(40)	15	10	0	−5	−15

Do not exercise out of doors when the wind chill factor is below the level indicated to the left of the heavy line.

*Metric equivalents are approximate.

Source: Adapted from a chart by Dr. Charles Egan.

APPENDIX E: FITNESS FOR SPORTS

You need to be fit to take part in games and sports. A good guide to your cardiovascular ability to participate is the level of your performance on the training tables.*

To participate in:

Sport

You need to be able to walk/jog 3 miles (4.8 km) in:

	(min.)
Archery	60-57
Badminton — social	39
— more vigorously	30-24
Basketball — recreational	39
— game	30-24
Bowling	54
Canoeing — leisurely	60-54
— vigorously	45-36
Cycling — 8 mph	60
— 10 mph	45
— 12 mph	36
— 10 mph	30
Gardening — raking	72
— mowing	42
— digging	36
Golf — using power cart	60
— pulling a club cart	48
— carrying clubs	42
Handball — easy	36
— more vigorously	30
Field hockey	30
Horseback riding — walking	60
— trotting	42
— galloping	33
Ice skating — leisurely	45
— quickly	36-30

Appendix E (cont'd.)

To participate in:	You need to be able to walk/jog 3 miles (4.8 km) in:
Sport	

	(min.)
Skiing — cross country (very leisurely)	42-36
— cross country (4 mph)	33
— cross country (5 mph)	30
— cross country (8 mph)	21
— downhill (easily)	42-36
— downhill (vigorously)	36-30
Snowshoeing	30-24
Soccer	54-36
	(depending on position and level of play)
Squash	25-18
Swimming (assuming a reasonably proficient swimmer, and optimal water temperature of 82-86°F [28-30°C])	
Breast stroke	30-27
Crawl stroke	33-30
Back stroke	33-30
Side stroke	36-33
Treading water	60-54
Tennis — doubles	48
— singles	33

*Values are based on a 150-lb (70-kg) person.

APPENDIX F: PAR-Q AND YOU

The Physical Activity Readiness Questionnaire (PAR-Q) is designed to help you help yourself. Many health benefits are associated with regular exercise, and the completion of PAR-Q is a sensible first step to take if you are planning to increase the amount of physical activity in your life.

For most people physical activity should not pose any problem or hazard. PAR-Q has been designed to identify the small number of adults for whom physical activity might be inappropriate or those who should have medical advice concerning the type of activity most suitable for them.

Common sense is your best guide in answering these few questions. Please read them carefully and check (✓) the ☐ YES or ☐ NO opposite the question if it applies to you.

Yes	No	
☐	☐	1. Has a doctor ever said that you have a heart condition and recommended only medically supervised activity?
☐	☐	2. Do you have chest pain brought on by physical activity?
☐	☐	3. Have you developed chest pain in the past month?
☐	☐	4. Do you tend to lose consciousness or fall over as a result of dizziness?
☐	☐	5. Do you have a bone or joint problem that could be aggravated by the proposed physical activity?
☐	☐	6. Has a doctor ever recommended medication for your blood pressure or a heart condition?
☐	☐	7. Are you aware through your own experience, or a doctor's advice, of any other physical reason against your exercising without medical supervision?

Note: If you have a temporary illness, such as a common cold, or are not feeling well at this time — **postpone.**

Appendix F (cont'd.)

If you answered YES to one or more questions

If you have not recently done so, consult your personal physician by telephone or in person BEFORE increasing your physical activity and/or taking a fitness appraisal. Tell your physician what questions you answered YES to on PAR-Q or present your PAR-Q copy.

Programs

After medical evaluation, seek advice from your physician as to your suitability for:
- unrestricted physical activity starting off easily and progressing gradually
- restricted or supervised activity to meet your specific needs, at least on an initial basis. Check in your community for special programs or services.

If you answered NO to all questions

If you answered PAR-Q accurately, you have reasonable assurance of your present suitability for:
- A GRADUATED EXERCISE PROGRAM — a gradual increase in proper exercise promotes good fitness development while minimizing or eliminating discomfort.
- A FITNESS APPRAISAL — the Canadian Standardized Test of Fitness (CSTF).

Postpone

If you have a temporary minor illness, such as a common cold.

Revised Physical Activity Readiness Questionnaire (PAR-Q). PAR-Q Validation Report. British Columbia Ministry of Health/Produced by the British Columbia Ministry of Health and the Department of National Health & Welfare. From **Canadian Standardized Test of Fitness (CSTF) Operations Manual**, 3rd Ed. With the permission of Fitness Canada, Fitness and Amateur Sport Canada, Ottawa, 1986.

APPENDIX G: HOW TO ESTIMATE YOUR RATE OF STEPPING

How to Estimate Your Rate of Stepping, the Resulting Energy Cost, and Target Heart Rate from Your Weight and Age

Rate of Stepping (steps per min.)	Energy Cost of Stepping (milliliters of oxygen)

MALE

Weight lbs. (kg.) / AGE	110 (49.9)	120 (54.4)	130 (59.0)	140 (63.5)	150 (68.0)	160 (72.6)	170 (77.1)	180 (81.6)	190 (86.2)	200 (90.7)	210 (95.3)	220 (99.8)
20-29	120 / 1570	120 / 1690	120 / 1813	126 / 2018	126 / 2143	126 / 2273	126 / 2398	126 / 2524	126 / 2653	126 / 2779	126 / 2908	126 / 3034
30-39	108 / 1437	114 / 1618	114 / 1734	114 / 1848	114 / 1962	114 / 2079	114 / 2192	114 / 2307	114 / 2423	120 / 2658	120 / 2781	120 / 2901
40-49	96 / 1304	96 / 1400	96 / 1498	102 / 1679	102 / 1781	102 / 1885	102 / 1987	102 / 2089	102 / 2193	102 / 2295	102 / 2400	102 / 2502
50-60	78 / 1105	78 / 1183	78 / 1262	78 / 1340	78 / 1418	78 / 1498	84 / 1679	84 / 1763	84 / 1849	84 / 1933	84 / 2018	84 / 2103

FEMALE

Weight lbs. (kg.) / AGE	80 (36.3)	90 (40.8)	100 (45.4)	110 (49.9)	120 (54.4)	130 (59.0)	140 (63.5)	150 (68.0)	160 (72.6)	170 (77.1)	180 (81.6)	190 (86.2)
20-29	96 / 974	102 / 1125	102 / 1229	102 / 1331	102 / 1433	108 / 1616	108 / 1724	108 / 1832	108 / 1942	108 / 2050	108 / 2158	108 / 2268
30-39	96 / 974	96 / 1070	102 / 1229	102 / 1331	102 / 1433	102 / 1537	102 / 1639	108 / 1832	108 / 1942	108 / 2050	108 / 2158	108 / 2268
40-49	84 / 877	84 / 961	84 / 1047	90 / 1198	90 / 1288	90 / 1380	90 / 1469	90 / 1560	90 / 1652	90 / 1742	96 / 1288	96 / 2038
50-60	60 / 684	60 / 744	60 / 805	60 / 865	60 / 925	60 / 986	60 / 1046	60 / 1106	60 / 1168	60 / 1228	60 / 1288	60 / 1349

Appendix G (cont'd.)

Target Heart Rates
(age-related) after 3-5 minutes of stepping

Age (Years)	Heart Rate (Beats/min.)
20-30	160/min.
30-40	150/min.
40-50	140/min.
50-60	130/min.
60-70	120/min.

APPENDIX H:

Cholesterol Screening and Treatment Guidelines Age: 30 years and over (Adapted from NCEP Report, 1988)		

Level	Blood Cholesterol	Risk	Action
1	Less than 200 mg/dL (5.2 mmol/L)	Desirable	Recheck within 5 years.
2	200–240 mg/dL (5.2–6.2 mmol/L)	Borderline High	
	2a *Without CHD or two other risk factors*[1], goal is to keep total cholesterol below 240 mg/dL (6.2 mmol/L); LDL-cholesterol below 160 mg/dL (4.1 mmol/L); and HDL-cholesterol above 35 mg/dL (0.9 mmol/L).		Restrict saturated fats; recheck total cholesterol in 1 year. Maintain less than 240 mg/dL (6.2 mmol/L).
	2b With CHD or two other risk factors, goal is to keep total cholesterol below 200 mg/dL (5.2 mmol/L); LDL-C below 130 mg/dL (3.4 mmol/L); and HDL-C above 35 mg/dL (0.9 mmol/L).	High Risk	Check triglycerides, LDL and HDL-cholesterol.[2] If abnormal, Step I of AHA diet.[3] Check blood fats again at 6 and 12 weeks. Once goal is attained, maintain diet, check blood cholesterol after 3 months for first year, then 6-monthly thereafter. *If goal is not attained*, Step II of AHA diet.[3] Check blood cholesterol at 6 and 12 weeks. If goal still not attained, physician may consider drug therapy.
3	Greater than 240 mg/dL (6.2 mmol/L; with or without CHD risk factors, goal is to keep cholesterol below 200 mg/dL (5.2 mmol/L); LDL-C below 130 mg/dL (3.4 mmol/L); and HDL-C above 35 mg/dL (0.9 mmol/L).	High Risk	As for 2b, although some physicians may wish to go straight to Step II diet, or in presence of CHD, to drug therapy.

Appendix H (cont'd.)

---

[1]**Risk Factors**
- male gender
- family history of CHD (heart attack or sudden death before age 55 years in parent or sibling)
- cigarette smoking
- hypertension
- diabetes
- history of stroke
- severe obesity (30% overweight)

---

[2]**LDL-Cholesterol:** How to calculate your LDL-cholesterol

$$LDL-C = T-CHOL - [Trig + 5 - HDL-C] \text{ (mg/dL)}$$
$$LDL-C = T-CHOL - [Trig + 2.2 - HDL-C] \text{ (mmol/L)}$$

Less than 130 mg/dL (3.4 mmol/L)	Desirable
130 - 160 mg/dL (3.4 mmol/L)	Borderline Risk
160 + mg/dL (4.2 + mmol/L	High Risk

***HDL-Cholesterol:** Greater than 35 mg/dL (0.9 mmol/L)   Desirable (the higher the better)

* *You will notice that the ratio of total cholesterol to HDL-cholesterol is not mentioned in the screening guide, although in recent data it is emerging as having a highly significant inverse relationship with CHD and a better indicator than either total cholesterol or HDL-cholesterol as isolated measures.*

RATIO (TC to HDL-C)

Women	Men	Risk
2.5	3.4	1/2 average
4.4	5.1	average
6.4	6.8	2X average
7.5	7.8	3X average

---

[3]**The American Heart Association Recommended Low-Fat Diet:**

Nutrient	Recommended Intake	
	Step I Diet	**Step II Diet**
Total Fat	Less than 30% of Total Calories	
Saturated Fatty Acids	Less than 10% of Total Calories	Less than 7% of Total Calories
Polyunsaturated Fatty Acids	Up to 10% of Total Calories	
Monounsaturated Fatty Acids	10 to 15% of Total Calories	
Carbohydrates	50 to 60% of Total Calories	
Protein	10 to 20% of Total Calories	
Cholesterol	Less than 300 mg/day	Less than 200 mg/day
Total Calories	To achieve and maintain desirable weight	

Bibliography

Antiplatelet Trialists' Collaboration. "Secondary prevention of vascular disease by prolonged antiplatelet treatment." *British Medical Journal*, 296:320, 1988.

Barrett-Connor E, Wingard D. "Sex differential in ischemic heart disease mortality in diabetics: a prospective population-based study." *American Journal of Epidemiology*, 118:489-496, 1983.

Blair SN, Kohl HW, Paffenbarger RS Jr, et al. "Physical fitness and all-cause mortality: a prospective study of healthy men and women." *Journal of the American Medical Association*, 262:2395-2401, 1989.

Blair SN, Goodyear NN, Gibbons LW, Cooper KH. "Physical fitness and incidence of hypertension in healthy normotensive men and women." *Journal of the American Medical Association*, 252:487-490, 1984.

Blankenhorn DH, Nessim SA, Johnson RL, et al. "Beneficial effects of combined colestipol-niacin therapy on coronary atherosclerosis and coronary venous bypass grafts." *Journal of the American Medical Association*, 257:3233-3240, 1987.

Brown MS, Goldstein JL. "A receptor mediated pathway for cholesterol homeostasis." *Science*, 232:34-47, 1986.

Campeau L, Enjalbert M, Lesperance J, et al. "The relation of risk factors to the development of atherosclerosis in saphenous-vein bypass grafts and the progression of disease in the native circulation." *New England Journal of Medicine*, 21:1329-32, 1984.

Coronary Drug Project Research Group. "Factors influencing long-term prognosis after recovery from myocardial infarction. Three-year findings of the Coronary Drug Project." *Journal of Chronic Diseases*, 27:267, 1974.

The Coronary Drug Project Research Group. "Clofibrate and niacin in coronary heart disease." *Journal of the American Medical Association*, 231:360-381, 1975.

Council on Scientific Affairs, American Medical Association. "Physician-supervised exercise programs in rehabilitation of patients with coronary heart disease." *Journal of the American Medical Association*, 245:1463-66, 1981.

Croft P, Hannaford PC. "Risk factors for acute myocardial infarction in women: evidence from the Royal College of General Practitioners' Oral Contraception Study." *British Medical Journal*, 298:165-168, 1989.

Davidson MH, Dugan LD, Burns JH, Bova J, Story K, Drennan KB. "The hypocholesterolemic effects of a-glucan in oatmeal and oat bran. A dose-controlled study." *Journal of the American Medical Association*, 265:1833-1839, 1991.

Dimsdale JE. "A perspective on Type A behavior and coronary disease" (editorial). *New England Journal of Medicine*, 318:110-112, 1988.

Doll R, Peto R. "Mortality in relation to smoking: twenty years' observations of British doctors." *British Medical Journal*, 4:1525, 1976.

Dyerberg J, Bang HO. "Haemostatic function and platelet polyunsaturated fatty acids in Eskimos." *Lancet*, ii:433-435, 1979.

Ekelund LG, Haskell, WL, Johnson JL, et al. "Physical fitness as a predictor of cardiovascular mortality in asymptomatic North American men." The Lipid Research Clinic's Mortality Follow-up Study. *New England Journal of Medicine*, 319:1379-84, 1988.

Enig MG. "Health and physiological effects of dietary trans fatty acids." A summary report from the University of Maryland Lipids Research Group. Department of Chemistry and Biochemistry, College Park, Maryland, December 1988.

Frick MH, Elo O, Haapa K, et al. "Helsinki Heart Study: Primary prevention trial with gemfibrozil in middle-aged men with dyslipidemia." *New England Journal of Medicine*, 317:1237-1245, 1987.

Frisch RE, Wyshak G, Albright TE, Albright NL, Schiff I. "Lower prevalence of diabetes in female former college athletes compared with nonathletes." *Diabetes*, 35:1101-1105, 1986.

Hagberg J. "Exercise, fitness, and hypertension." Bouchard et al, eds. *Exercise, fitness and health: a consensus of current knowledge*. Champaign: Human Kinetics Books, 1990.

Hegele R, Emi M, Lily L, Hopkins P, Williams R, Lalouel J. "Clinical applications of DNA markers in a Utah family with hypercholesterolemia." *American Journal of Cardiology*, 63:109-112, 1989.

Hole DJ, Gillis CR, Chopra CR, Hawthorne VM. "Passive smoking and cardiorespiratory health in a general population in the west of Scotland." *British Medical Journal*, 299:423-427, 1989.

Holmes T, Rahe R. "The social readjustment rating scale." *Journal of Psychosomatic Research*, 11:213-18, 1967.

Hypertension Detection and Follow-up Program Cooperative Group. "Presentation of 5-year results." Bethesda, MD: US Dept. of Health and Human Services, 1980.

Intersalt Cooperative Research Group. "Intersalt: an international study of electrolyte excretion and blood pressure. Results for 24 hour urinary sodium and potassium excretion." *British Medical Journal*, 297:319-328, 1988.

Kanner A, Coyne J, Schaefer C, et al. "Comparison of two modes of stress measurement: daily hassles and uplifts versus major life events." *Journal of Behavioral Medicine*, 4:1-39, 1981.

Kavanagh T. "Evidence to date for the beneficial effect of exercise following myocardial infarction." Mathes P, Halhuber MJ, eds. *Controversies in Cardiac Rehabilitation*. Berlin: Springer-Verlag, 1982, pp 43-52.

————. "Exercise rehabilitation after coronary artery bypass graft surgery." Yacoub M, ed. *Annual of Cardiac Surgery 1987*. Gower Academic Journals, 1987, pp 140-43.

————. "Exercise and coronary artery disease." Basmajian JV, ed. *Therapeutic Exercise*, 4th edition. Baltimore: Williams and Wilkins, 1984, pp 565-586.

————. "Exercise rehabilitation after heart transplantation." Kapoor AS, Laks H, Schroeder JS, Yacoub M, eds. *Cardiomyopathies and Heart-Lung Transplantation*. Los Angeles: McGraw-Hill, 1991, pp 359-368.

————. "Exercise and therapy of the cardiac transplant patient." Miller HS, ed. *Exercise and the Heart in Health and Cardiac Disease*. New York: Marcel Dekker, Inc., 1991.

————, Yacoub M. "The benefits of exercise for heart transplant patients." *Perspectives in Cardiology*, 4(1):21-37, 1988.

————. "The Toronto Rehabilitation Centre's cardiac exercise program." *Journal of Cardiopulmonary Rehabilitation*, 2:496-502, 1982.

————. "Exercise rehabilitation after coronary artery bypass graft surgery." *Current Opinion in Cardiology*, 4:807-811, 1989.

————, Mertens DJ, Baigrie RS, et al. "Assessment of patients with clinical congestive heart failure: ventilatory threshold or aerobic power determination?" *Sports Medicine Training and Rehabilitation*, 3:37-48, 1991.

————, Matosevic V. "Cardiac rehabilitation for return to work." *Journal of Occupational Health and Safety*, 5(3):213-220, 1989.

——— , Shephard RJ, Pandit V. "Marathon running after myocardial infarction." *Journal of the American Medical Association*, 229(12):1602-05, 1974.

——— , Shephard RJ, Chisholm A, et al. "Prognostic indexes for patients with ischemic heart disease enrolled in an exercise-centered rehabilitation program." *American Journal of Cardiology*, 44:1230-40, 1979.

——— , Yacoub MH, Mertens DJ, Kennedy J, Campbell RB, Sawyer P. "Cardiorespiratory responses to exercise training after orthotopic cardiac transplantation." *Circulation*, 77:162-171, 1988.

——— , Yacoub MH, Mertens DJ, et al. "Exercise rehabilitation after heterotopic cardiac transplantation." *Journal of Cardiopulmonary Rehabilitation*, 9:303-310, 1989.

——— , Yacoub MH, Campbell R, Mertens D. "Marathon running after cardiac transplantation: a case history." *Journal of Cardiopulmonary Rehabilitation*, 6:16, 1986.

Keys A. "Coronary heart disease in seven countries." *Circulation*, 1(sup):41-42, 1970.

——— , Anderson JT, Grande F. "Serum cholesterol response to changes in the diet. IV. Particular saturated fatty acids in the diet." *Metabolism*, 14:776, 1965c.

Kromhout D, Bosschieter EB, de Lezene Coulander C. "The inverse relationship between fish consumption and 20-year mortality from coronary heart disease." *New England Journal of Medicine*, 312:1205-1209, 1985.

Krueger DE, Ellenberg SS, Bloom S, et al. "Risk factors for fatal heart attack in young women." *American Journal of Epidemiology*, 113:357-370, 1981.

Leon AS, Connett J, Jacobs DR, et al. "Leisure-time physical activity levels and the risk of coronary heart disease and death." *Journal of the American Medical Association*, 258:2388-2395, 1987.

Lipid Research Clinics Program. "The Lipid Research Clinics Coronary Primary Prevention Trial Results. I. Reduction in incidence of coronary heart disease." *Journal of the American Medical Association*, 241:351, 1984a.

——— . "The Lipid Research Clinics Coronary Primary Prevention Trial results. II. The Relationship of reduction in incidence of coronary heart disease to cholesterol lowering." *Journal of the American Medical Association*, 251:365, 1984b.

Mann JI, Doll R, Thorogood M, et al. "Risk factors for myocardial infarction in young women." *British Journal of Preventive Medicine*, 30:94-100, 1976.

Marmot MG, Syme SL, Kagan A, et al. "Epidemiologic studies of CHD and stroke in Japanese men living in Japan, Hawaii and California. Prevalence of coronary and hypertensive heart disease and associated risk factors." *American Journal of Epidemiology*, 102:514, 1975.

May GS, Eberlein KA, Furberg CD, Passamani ER, DeMets DL. "Secondary prevention after myocardial infarction: a review of long-term trials." *Progress in Cardiovascular Disease*, 24:331-352, 1982.

Medical Research Council Working Party. "MRC trial of treatment of mild hypertension: principal results." *British Medical Journal*, 291:97-104, 1985.

Morris JN, Heady JA, Raffle PAB, et al. "Coronary heart-disease and physical activity of work." *Lancet*, 2:1053-57, 1953.

——— , Everitt MG, Pollard R, et al. "Vigorous exercise in leisure-time: protection against coronary heart disease." *Lancet*, 2:1207-10, 1980.

Multiple Risk Factor Intervention Trial Group. "Multiple Risk Factor Intervention Trial: Risk factor change and mortality results." *Journal of the American Medical Association*, 248:1465-1477, 1982.

National Cholesterol Education Program. "Report of the Expert Panel on Detection, Evaluation, and Treatment of High Blood Cholesterol in Adults." National Institutes of Health Publication, No. 88-2925, January 1988.

O'Connor GT, Buring JE, Yusuf S, et al. "An overview of randomized trials of rehabilitation with exercise after myocardial infarction." *Circulation*, 80:234-244, 1989.

Oldridge NB, Guyatt GH, Fischer ME, Rimm Aa. "Cardiac rehabilitation after myocardial infarction: combined experience of randomized clinical trials." *Journal of the American Medical Association*, 260:945-950, 1988.

Ornish D, Brown SE, Scherwitz LW, et al. "Can lifestyle changes reverse coronary heart disease?" *Lancet*, 326:129-133, 1990.

Paffenbarger RS Jr, Laughlin ME, Gima AS, et al. "Work activity of longshoremen as related to death from coronary heart disease and stroke." *New England Journal of Medicine*, 282:1109-1114, 1970.

———, Hyde RT, Wing AL, et al. "Physical activity, all-cause mortality and longevity of college alumni." *New England Journal of Medicine*, 314:605-613, 1986.

Peto R, Gray R, Collins R, et al. "Randomised trial of prophylactic daily aspirin in British male doctors." *British Medical Journal*, 296:313-316, 1988.

Powell KE, Thompson PD, Caspersen CJ, Kendrick JS. "Physical activity and the incidence of coronary heart disease." *Annual Review of Public Health*, 8:253-287, 1987.

Puska P, Tuomilehto J, Salonen J, et al. "Changes in coronary risk factors during comprehensive five-year community programme to control cardiovascular diseases (North Karelia project)." *British Medical Journal*, 2:1173-1178, 1979.

Ragland DR, Brand RJ. "Type A behaviour and mortality from coronary heart disease." *New England Journal of Medicine*, 318:65-69, 1988.

Rosenberg L, Miller DR, Kaufman DW, et al. "Myocardial infarction in women under 50 years of age." *Journal of the American Medical Association*, 250:2801-06, 1983.

Selye H. *The Stress of Life*. New York: McGraw-Hill, 1956.

Shephard RJ, Corey P, Kavanagh T. "Exercise compliance and the prevention of a recurrence of myocardial infarction." *Medicine Science Sports and Exercise*, 13(1):1-5, 1981.

Siscovick DS, Weiss NS, Fletcher RH, et al. "The incidence of primary cardiac arrest during vigorous exercise." *New England Journal of Medicine*, 311:874-77, 1984.

Slattery ML, Jacobs DR Jr, Nichaman MZ. "Leisure time physical activity and coronary heart disease death. The US railroad study." *Circulation*, 79:304-311, 1989.

Stampfer MJ, Colditz GA, Willett WC, et al. "Postmenopausal estrogen therapy and cardiovascular disease. Ten-year follow-up from the Nurses' Health Study." *New England Journal of Medicine*, 325:756-762, 1991.

Steering committee of the Physicians' Health Study Research Group. "Preliminary report: findings from the aspirin component of the ongoing physicians' health study." *New England Journal of Medicine*, 318:262-264, 1988.

Steingart RM, Packer M, Hamm P, et al. "Sex differences in the management of coronary artery disease." *New England Journal of Medicine*, 325:226-230, 1991.

Stratton JR, Chandler WL, Schwartz RS, et al. "Effects of physical conditioning on fibrinolytic variables and fibrinogen in young and old healthy adults." *Circulation*, 83:1692-1697, 1991.

Takekoshi H, Matsuoka K, Suzuki Y, et al. "A ten year follow up study in NIDDM with or without exercise." Vannasaeng S, Nitiyanant W, Chandrapasert S, eds. *Proceedings of the International Symposium on Epidemiology of Diabetes Mellitus, Bangkok, 1987*, pp 149-152.

Thompson PD, Funk EJ, Carleton RA, Sturner WQ. "Incidence of death during jogging in Rhode Island from 1975 through 1980." *Journal of the American Medical Association*, 247:2535-2538, 1982.

Turpeinen O, Karvonen MJ, Pekkarinen M, et al. "Dietary prevention of coronary heart disease: The Finnish Mental Hospital Study." *International Journal of Epidemiology*, 8:99, 1979.

V.A. Cooperative Study Group on Antihypertensive Agents. "Effects of treatment on morbidity in hypertension. I. Results in patients with diastolic blood pressures averaging 115 through 129 mm Hg." *Journal of the American Medical Association*, 202:1028, 1967.

——— . "Effects of treatment on morbibity in hypertension. II. Results in patients with diastolic blood pressure averaging 90 through 114 mm Hg." *Journal of the American Medical Association*, 213:1143, 1970.

W.H.O. Committee of Principal Investigators. "Clofibrate Trial: a cooperative trial in the primary prevention of ischaemic heart disease using clofibrate." *British Medical Journal*, 40:1069-1118, 1978.

Zock Pl, Katan MB, Merkus MP, van Dusseldorp M, Harryvan JL. "Effect of a lipid-rich fraction from boiled coffee on serum cholesterol." *Lancet*, 335:1235-1237, 1990.

Index

Acebutolot, 136
ACE inhibitors, 145
  captopril, 146
  enalapril, 146
  lisinopril, 146
Acetylsalicylic acid. *See* Aspirin
acute myocardial infarction, 17-19
  see also Heart attack
Adalat. *See* Nifedipine
Aerobic exercise, types of:
  cross-country skiing, 194
  dancing, 198
  motorized treadmills, 196
  outdoor cycling, 192-93
  rope-skipping, 197-98
  rowing machines, 196
  stair-climbing machines, 198-99
  stationary cycling, 194-96
  step, 199
  swimming, 193-94
  walking and jogging, 192
  walking with hand-held weights,
    196-97
Aerobic fitness, 182, 183-91
  and exertion rate, 189-91
  heart rate and, 188-89
  and intensity of workout, 185-86
  oxygen intake and, 186-88
Aging, and hypertension, 50-51
Air travel, and the heart patient, 301-
  03
Alcohol consumption:
  and coronary heart disease, 288-89
  and hypertension, 52-53
Aldactazide. *See* Hydrochlorothiazide
Ambulatory electrocardiogram
  monitoring, 132
American Academy of Pediatrics, 59
American Dietary Association, 111
American Heart Association, 110
  Low Fat Diet, 111
  Step II Diet, 234
American Medical Joggers'
  Association, 172
American National Cholesterol
  Education Program (NCEP), 119-
  20
Anaerobic fitness, 183, 185
Anderson, Dr. James, 109-10
Anderson, Professor Terry, 88
Android fat distribution, 77
  and health risk, 77-78
Angina pectoris:
  cause of, 2

cold-induced, 276-78
and coronary arteries, 2, 16-17
and endurance fitness, 246-49, 263-
  64
and the exercise test, 127-30
interval training, 264
nitrates and, 134-35
and Rate Pressure Product, 230-31
relief of through exercise
  rehabilitation, 229-34
silent, 128, 229
as symptom of coronary heart
  disease, 2
in women, 20
Angioplasty. *See* Percutaneous
  transluminal coronary angioplasty
Angiotensin-converting enzyme
  inhibitors. *See* ACE inhibitors
Animal studies, showing effects of
  exercise training, 162-65
Anti-clotting drugs:
  aspirin, 138-41
  fibrinolytics, 142-43
  warfarin, 141-42
Anticoagulants. *See* Anti-clotting drugs
Aorta, of the heart, 9, 12, 15
Appestat, brain, 81
Aspirin, 138-41
Atenolol, 136
Atheroma. *See* Lesion, atherosclerotic
Atherosclerosis, 15
  as cause of stroke, 21
  causes of, 22-31
  first stage in development of, 26-27
  gender as a risk factor for, 32-41
  see also Coronary atherosclerosis
atrium, of the heart, 9
Atromid-S. *See* Clofibrate

Banting, Dr., 56
Bell Telephone Company, 70
Benefits of exercise rehabilitation:
  heart performance, 229
  psychological, 228-29
  relief of angina, 229-34
  retarding progression of coronary
    atherosclerosis, 234-35
  secondary prevention, 235-36
Benzinger Reflex, 268
Best, Dr., 56
Beta-adrenoreceptor-blocker. *See* Beta-
  blockers
Beta-blockers, 135-37, 230
  and endurance fitness, 249-50